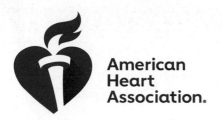

American
Heart
Association.

P9-DNU-570

STUDENT WORKBOOK

HEARTSAVER®

FIRST AID | CPR | AED

© 2021 American Heart Association
ISBN 978-1-61669-827-0
Printed in the United States of America

First American Heart Association Printing February 2021
10 9 8 7 6 5 4 3 2

i

Acknowledgments

The American Heart Association thanks the following people for their contributions to the development of this manual: Gustavo E. Flores, MD, NRP, FP-C; Eric Goralnick, MD, MS; and the AHA Heartsaver Project Team.

Contact Us

Contact the American Heart Association if you want more information on first aid, CPR, or AED training. You can visit **cpr.heart.org** or call 1-877-AHA-4CPR (877-242-4277) to find a class near you.

 To find out about any updates or corrections to this text, visit **heart.org/courseupdates**.

Contents

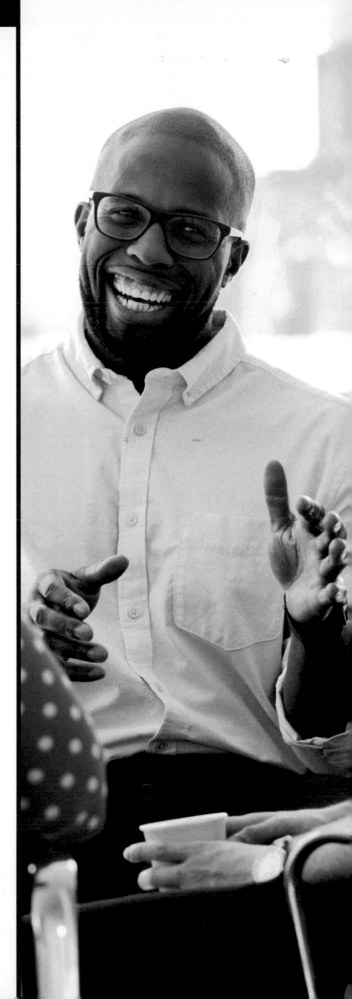

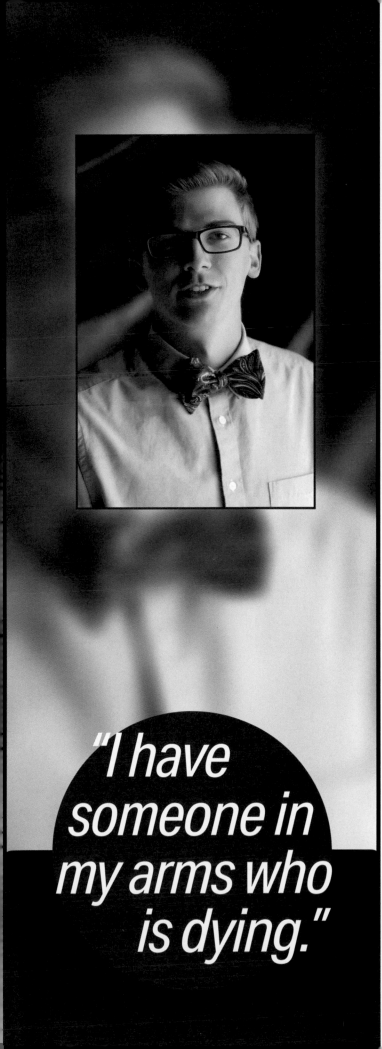

"I have someone in my arms who is dying."

Kurt's Story
Survivor's Story

It was early in my shift at the café, around 8:45 on a Monday morning, and I was still feeling tired and groggy. A customer ran up to the counter and asked, "Does anyone know CPR?" A man had collapsed outside, on the patio.

Suddenly, I was wide awake.

I didn't have formal training in cardiopulmonary resuscitation—that's CPR—but I had learned some skills from the American Heart Association website and from Boy Scouts, when I was a kid. At first, I was nervous, but there was no time to waste—somebody needed help now.

Outside, the adrenaline kicked in like a shot of espresso, and I knew exactly what to do. The customer had collapsed in a patio chair. I'll never forget his face—it was as pale as a piece of paper. He wasn't breathing, moving, or responding.

While someone called 9-1-1, we lowered the man to the patio. I remember thinking, "I have someone in my arms who is dying." Another barista held the man's head, and I started CPR. I put both hands on the center of his chest and just started pushing, hard and fast. I kept doing chest compressions and breaths for about 2 minutes, until medical help arrived.

After medical help took over, I washed up, tied my apron on, and went back to serving coffee. But for the rest of my shift, I wondered how that customer was doing.

Later, I found out he was a 66-year-old man named Mike. He survived his cardiac arrest and is doing well. I also found out that most people who witness a cardiac arrest either don't know CPR or are afraid to do it. So, they call 9-1-1—and then they wait. Medical help gets there as fast as they can, but in the United States, it still takes an average of 4 to 10 minutes for them to reach someone in cardiac arrest. The problem is, when someone's heart stops, death occurs within 10 minutes. That means receiving CPR from a bystander is a person's only chance to survive until medical help arrives. It also means any CPR is better than no CPR.

My career goal is to become an emergency medical technician and do search and rescue. But you don't have to be a medical professional to help save a life. By learning CPR, you too can be ready to help someone in cardiac arrest. It might even be a friend or a family member whose life is in your hands.

On your next coffee break, why not take the time to learn CPR?

What You Will Learn in This Course

Welcome to the Heartsaver® First Aid CPR AED Course. During this course, you will gain knowledge and skills that may help save a life. But the most important goal of this course is to teach you to act in an emergency. Sometimes, people don't act because they are afraid of doing the wrong thing. Recognizing that something is wrong and phoning 9-1-1 for help are the most important things you can do.

We'll also teach you how to keep yourself safe by assessing the scene *and* using personal protective equipment (PPE). And we'll discuss Good Samaritan laws, which protect first aid rescuers.

This book contains all the information that you need to understand and perform lifesaving CPR and first aid skills correctly. During the course, you will practice these skills and receive valuable coaching from your instructor.

The video in the course will cover many, but not all, of the skills in this workbook. So, to be fully prepared to help in an emergency, it is important to read this book before your class and regularly refer to it as a resource.

Successful Course Completion

During the course, you will be asked to practice and demonstrate important skills. As you read and study this workbook, pay attention to those skills.

If you complete all course requirements and demonstrate the skills correctly, you'll receive a course completion card. Your course completion card is valid for 2 years.

CPR AED Course Objectives*

At the end of the CPR AED portion of this course, you will be able to

- Describe how high-quality CPR improves survival
- Explain the concept of the Chain of Survival
- Recognize when someone needs CPR
- Describe how to perform CPR with help from others
- Demonstrate giving effective breaths by using mouth to mouth or a mask for all ages
- Demonstrate performing high-quality CPR for an adult, a child, and an infant
- Demonstrate using an AED on an adult and on a child
- Describe when and how to help a choking adult or child
- Demonstrate how to help a choking infant

*Course objectives may vary on the basis of the course topics taught.

First Aid Course Objectives*

This course also includes first aid. At the end of the first aid portion, you will be able to

- List the priorities, roles, and responsibilities of first aid rescuers
- Describe the key steps in first aid
- Demonstrate removing protective gloves
- Demonstrate finding the problem
- Describe the assessment and first aid actions for these life-threatening conditions: heart attack, difficulty breathing, choking, severe bleeding, shock, and stroke
- Describe when and how to help a choking adult, child, or infant

- Demonstrate how to help a choking infant
- Demonstrate how to use an epinephrine pen
- Demonstrate how to control bleeding and apply bandaging
- Recognize elements of common illnesses and injuries
- Describe the benefits of living a healthy lifestyle and the risks of smoking and vaping
- Describe how to find information on preventing illness and injury
- Recognize the legal questions that apply to first aid rescuers

*Course objectives may vary on the basis of the course topics taught.

Heartsaver Terms and Concepts

The following key terms and concepts are used throughout this course:

First Aid

First aid is the immediate care that you give a person with an illness or injury before rescuers with more advanced training arrive and take over.

Anyone, in any situation, can start giving first aid. It may help an ill or injured person recover more completely or more quickly. In serious emergencies, first aid can mean the difference between life and death.

Most often, you'll give first aid for minor illnesses or injuries. But you may also give first aid for problems that could become life threatening, such as providing aid for a heart attack, applying a tourniquet for severe bleeding, or giving epinephrine for a severe allergic reaction.

Preventing Illness and Injury

Being able to see an accident coming and helping to prevent illness and injury are important parts of your role as a first aid rescuer.

Responsive vs Unresponsive

During an emergency, the person you are helping might become unresponsive. Here is how to decide whether someone is responsive or unresponsive:

- *Responsive:* A person who is responsive will move, speak, blink, or otherwise react to you when you tap them and ask, "Are you OK?"
- *Unresponsive:* A person who does not move, speak, blink, or otherwise react is unresponsive.

For someone who is unresponsive, you will learn to check to see if that person needs CPR.

Agonal Gasps

A person in cardiac arrest will not be breathing normally or may only be gasping. When we refer to *gasps,* we mean agonal gasps. Agonal gasps are frequently present in the first minutes after cardiac arrest.

Someone who is gasping will seem to be drawing air in very quickly and may even move their mouth, jaw, head, or neck. The gasp may sound like a snort, snore, or groan. These gasps may appear forceful or weak. Some time may pass between gasps because they often happen at a slow rate.

Gasping is not regular or normal breathing. It's a sign of cardiac arrest in someone who is unresponsive.

Cardiopulmonary Resuscitation

CPR stands for cardiopulmonary resuscitation. When a person's heart stops suddenly, receiving CPR can double or even triple the chances of survival.

CPR is made up of 2 skills:

- Providing compressions
- Giving breaths

A *compression* is the act of pushing down hard and fast on the chest. When you push on the chest, you pump blood to the brain and other organs. To give CPR, you provide sets of 30 compressions and 2 breaths.

Automated External Defibrillator

AED stands for automated external defibrillator. It's a lightweight, portable device used to detect abnormal cardiac rhythms that require treatment. An AED can deliver an electrical shock to convert the rhythm back to normal.

When you give first aid, you will need to get the first aid kit and sometimes an AED. AEDs should be located in a building's main office, high-traffic area, or break room or in a high-risk area, such as a gym—anywhere that the most people can see and access them in an emergency.

Always find out the location of the nearest first aid kit and AED so that you can provide the best possible help if someone is ill or injured.

Adults, Children, and Infants

In this course, we use the following age definitions:

- **Adult:** Adolescent (after the onset of puberty) and older
- **Child:** 1 year of age to puberty
- **Infant:** Less than 1 year of age

Signs of puberty include chest or underarm hair on boys and any breast development for girls.

Treat anyone who has signs of puberty as an adult. If you are not sure whether someone is an adult or a child, provide emergency care as if the person is an adult.

Phone 9-1-1

In this course, we say, "phone 9-1-1." You may have a different emergency response number. If you do, phone your emergency response number instead of 9-1-1.

In an emergency, use the most readily available phone. This may be your own cell phone or the cell phone of someone who comes to help. After phoning 9-1-1, put the phone on speaker mode, if possible, so that the person providing emergency care can talk to the dispatcher.

Course Delivery and Options

This course will help prepare you for the most common types of first aid emergencies and equip you with CPR skills for adults, children, and infants. As part of Heartsaver First Aid CPR AED, the American Heart Association (AHA) designed a course that is flexible in its delivery, with the most current relevant science and information. It includes core concepts that you will be required to complete. In addition to these topics, your instructor may include optional topics. Check with your respective agency or workplace to ensure that the course or course path fulfills their requirements.

- **Heartsaver** is designed to be flexible for students who need to review only certain topics to meet requirements for the Heartsaver First Aid CPR AED Course. Course objectives may vary on the basis of the course topics taught.
- **Heartsaver Total** is designed to meet licensing requirements for Occupational Safety and Health Administration (OSHA) and other regulatory agencies.

In addition to the Heartsaver and Heartsaver Total course options, this course may be realigned to meet the needs of many audiences. Heartsaver First Aid CPR AED is designed to allow instructors the flexibility to target specific audience needs.

If you are a teacher or an office worker, your instructor may create an agenda that will be more targeted toward your first aid and CPR AED needs. For more information on those specific path topics, refer to Table 1.

Table 1. Topic List for Course and Path Options*

Topic	Heartsaver	Heartsaver Total	Office	Educator
			Recommended topics for these paths	
Introduction (for all)	✓	✓	✓	✓
CPR and AED Use for Adults[†]	✓	✓	✓	✓
CPR and AED Use for Children[†]	Optional	Optional	Optional	✓
CPR for Infants[†]	Optional	Optional	Optional	Optional
How to Help an Adult With a Drug Overdose Emergency	Optional	✓	Optional	Optional
Water Safety	Optional	✓	Optional	Optional
Duties, Roles, and Responsibilities of First Aid Rescuers (finding the problem[†]**)**	✓	✓	✓	✓
Personal Safety (exposure to blood and removing gloves[†]**)**	✓	✓	✓	✓
Breathing Problems (Asthma)	Optional	✓	Optional	Optional
Choking in an Adult, a Child, or an Infant	Optional	✓	Optional	Optional

(continued)

Topic	Heartsaver	Heartsaver Total	Office	Educator
			Recommended topics for these paths	
Allergic Reactions (using an epinephrine pen†)	✓	✓	✓	✓
Heart Attack	✓	✓	✓	✓
Fainting	Optional	✓	Optional	Optional
Diabetes and Low Blood Sugar	Optional	✓	✓	✓
Stroke	✓	✓	✓	✓
Seizure	Optional	✓	✓	✓
External Bleeding (direct pressure and bandaging† and tourniquet)	✓	✓	✓	✓
Shock	Optional	✓	Optional	Optional
Wounds (Bleeding From the Nose, Bleeding From the Mouth, Tooth Injuries, and Eye Injuries)	Optional	✓	✓	✓
Penetrating and Puncturing Injuries	Optional	✓	✓	✓
Amputation	Optional	✓	✓	✓
Internal Bleeding	Optional	✓	✓	✓
Concussions	Optional	✓	Optional	✓
Head, Neck, and Spine Injuries	Optional	✓	✓	✓
Broken Bones and Sprains	Optional	✓	Optional	✓
Splinting	Optional	✓	Optional	✓
Burns and Electrical Injuries	Optional	✓	Optional	✓
Bites and Stings	Optional	✓	Optional	✓
Heat-Related Emergencies	Optional	✓	Optional	✓
Cold-Related Emergencies	Optional	✓	Optional	✓
Poison Emergencies	Optional	✓	Optional	✓
Risks of Smoking and Vaping	Optional	✓	Optional	Optional
Benefits of a Healthy Lifestyle	Optional	✓	Optional	✓
Preventing Illness and Injury	Optional	✓	✓	✓

*Topic groups vary by course or path.

†Topic requires a skills test.

Legal Concerns

Deciding to Provide First Aid

Providing first aid and CPR may be part of your job description. If so, you must help while you're working. However, when you're off duty, you can choose whether to provide first aid. If you choose to help, first ask if you can help. Anyone has the right to refuse your help.

Good Samaritan Laws

If you have legal questions about providing first aid, you should know that all states have Good Samaritan laws that protect anyone who gives first aid and CPR. The laws differ from state to state, so be sure to check the laws in your area or talk to your instructor.

Protecting the Person's Privacy

As a first aid rescuer, you may learn private things about the people you help, such as a medical condition. Give all information about an ill or injured person to EMS rescuers. If you are in your workplace, also give this information to your company's emergency response program supervisor. You may need to fill out a report for your company.

If an emergency does happen in your workplace, you must not share any information you learn with other coworkers. Keep private things private.

Have Confidence in Your Training

Thank you for taking the Heartsaver First Aid CPR AED Course. As a first aid rescuer, you can prevent further illness or injury, reduce suffering, and help someone heal faster—you might even save a life.

Refresh your knowledge by reviewing this book often, and keep the reference guide handy. Even if you don't remember all the steps exactly, it is important for you to try. Any help is better than no help at all. More than anything, we want you to have both the knowledge and the confidence to act in an emergency. Recognizing that something is wrong and getting help on the way is one of the most important things you can do.

We also want to recognize the heroes who step in to help save a life during an emergency. If you have a story to share or want to be inspired by other survivor stories, please visit **heart.org/heartsaverhero**.

Duties, Roles, and Responsibilities of First Aid Rescuers

Some people may be required to perform first aid while they are at work. For example, police officers, firefighters, flight attendants, lifeguards, teachers, and park rangers may have a duty to give first aid when they are working. Others may not have a duty to respond but want to know how to help their family members, friends, coworkers, and customers in the event of an emergency.

Your Role in the EMS System

Your role as a first aid rescuer is to
- Recognize that an emergency exists
- Make sure that the scene is safe for you and the ill or injured person
- Phone 9-1-1
- Provide care until someone with more advanced training arrives and takes over

When you phone 9-1-1, you activate a network of emergency responders, or emergency medical services (EMS). Getting help on the way quickly in an emergency can save a life.

Find the Problem

Before you give first aid, assess the ill or injured person to find out what the problem is. Sometimes the problem is apparent, and you can begin to give first aid. Other times, the problem may not be easily seen, and you will have to follow the below steps before providing first aid. They are listed in order of importance, with the most important step listed first.

Actions to Take: Find the Problem
- Make sure that the scene is safe.
- Check to see if the person responds. Approach the person, tap them, and shout, "Are you OK? Are you OK?" (Figure 1)

If the person is responsive

- Ask if you can help.
- If the person only moves, moans, or groans, shout for help. Phone or send someone else to phone 9-1-1 and get the first aid kit and an AED.
- Check for breathing.
  - If the person is breathing and doesn't need immediate first aid, look for any obvious signs of injury, such as bleeding, broken bones, burns, or bites.
  - Look for any medical information jewelry. It can tell you if the person has a serious medical condition (Figure 2).

(continued)

Actions to Take: Find the Problem *(continued)*

If the person is unresponsive

- Shout for help and phone 9-1-1.
  - Phone or send someone else to phone 9-1-1 and get a first aid kit and AED.
  - If you are alone and have a cell phone, put it on speaker mode and phone 9-1-1. Go get the first aid kit and AED yourself.
- Check for breathing.
  - If the person is breathing normally, stay with them until advanced help arrives. Check for injuries and medical information jewelry.
  - If the person is not breathing normally or is only gasping, begin CPR and use an AED (see the CPR and AED section).
- Stay with the person until advanced help arrives.

Figure 1. Check to see if the person is responsive or unresponsive. Tap and shout, "Are you OK?"

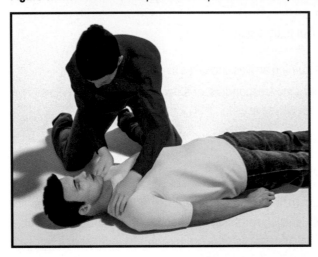

Figure 2. Look for medical information jewelry.

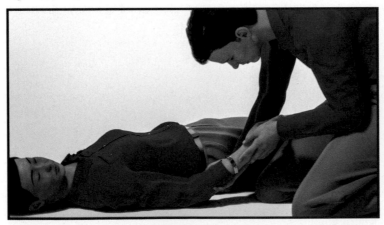
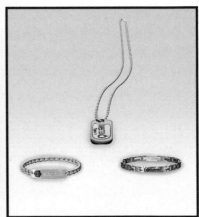

When to Phone 9-1-1

As you assess the need for first aid, it's important to know when and how to phone for help. Phoning 9-1-1 activates the EMS network of responders. Once you phone 9-1-1, the dispatcher—the person who answers 9-1-1 calls—will guide you in what to do until help arrives. People with advanced training (emergency medical technicians, paramedics, and others) usually arrive and take over soon after you call.

Make sure you know the nearest location of a phone to use in an emergency (Figure 3). In many workplaces, the first aid kit and AED are stored right by the emergency phone.

Figure 3. Know the location of the nearest phone to use in an emergency. You also should know where the first aid kit and AED are stored.

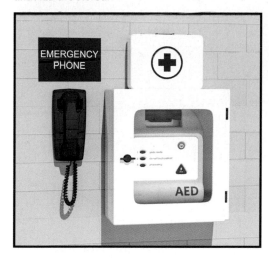

When to Phone for Help

Your company may have its own instructions about when you should phone the emergency response number (or 9-1-1).

As a rule, you should phone 9-1-1 and ask for help whenever someone is seriously ill or injured or you are not sure what to do in an emergency.

Some examples of when you should phone 9-1-1 are if the ill or injured person

- Doesn't respond to voice or touch
- Has chest discomfort (a sign of a possible heart attack)
- Shows signs of a stroke
- Has a problem breathing
- Is suspected of having a drug overdose
- Has a severe injury or burn
- Has severe bleeding
- Has a seizure
- Suddenly can't move a part of the body
- Received an electric shock
- Was exposed to poison

How to Phone for Help

It's also important for you to know how to phone for help from your location. Do you know how to activate the emergency response number in your workplace? For example, do you need to dial 9 for an outside line? Or is there an internal number to phone that will notify responders who are on-site? Write the emergency response number in this student workbook, in the first aid kit, and near the telephone.

Actions to Take: Phone for Help

If you are alone

- Shout for help.
- If no one answers and the person needs immediate care and you have a cell phone, phone 9-1-1 and put the phone on speaker mode.
- Listen to the dispatcher's instructions, such as how to give first aid, perform CPR, or use an AED.

If you are with others

- Stay with the ill or injured person and be ready to give first aid or CPR if you know how.
- Send someone else to phone 9-1-1 and get the first aid kit and AED if available.
- Have the person put the phone on speaker mode so that you can receive instructions from the dispatcher.

Follow the Dispatcher's Instructions

When you're on the phone with the dispatcher, don't hang up until the dispatcher tells you to. Answering the dispatcher's questions won't delay the arrival of help. Knowing the address of your location will help emergency responders reach you more quickly. That's why it's important to always be aware of your surroundings.

First Aid Kit Maintenance

One responsibility of a first aid provider is to maintain the first aid kit. The kit should always contain the supplies you'll need for most common emergencies.

Table 2 is a sample list of contents for a first aid kit. The list divides recommended first aid kit supplies into 2 categories: Class A and Class B. Class A kits are suitable for homes or smaller workplaces. Class B kits are for larger workplaces and are designed to treat injuries more often found in densely populated workplaces with complex or high-risk environments, such as warehouses, factories, and outdoor areas. Use your best judgment on which class is most suitable for your location, and always be sure to restock the kit after any emergency. These lists follow the standards of the American National Standards Institute (ANSI); you can find more information at **ansi.org**.

Table 2. Sample First Aid Kit List

First aid supply	Minimum quantity		Minimum size or volume	
	Class A kits	Class B kits	US	Metric
Adhesive bandage	16	50	1 × 3 in	2.5 × 7.5 cm
Adhesive tape	1	2	2.5 yd (total)	2.3 m
Antibiotic application	10	25	1/57 oz	0.5 g
Antiseptic	10	50	1/57 oz	0.5 g
Breathing barrier	1	1	N/A	N/A
Burn dressing (gel soaked)	1	2	4 × 4 in	10 × 10 cm
Burn treatment	10	25	1/32 oz	0.9 g
Cold pack	1	2	4 × 5 in	10 × 12.5 cm
Eye covering (with means of attachment)	2	2	2.9 sq in	19 sq cm
Eye/skin wash	1 fl oz total			29.6 mL
		4 fl oz total		118.3 mL
Hand sanitizer	6	10	1/32 oz	0.9 g
Medical exam gloves	2 pair	4 pair	N/A	N/A
Roller bandage (2 inch)	1	2	2 in × 4 yd	5 cm × 3.66 m
Roller bandage (4 inch)	0	1	4 in × 4 yd	10 cm × 3.66 m
Scissors	1	1	N/A	N/A
Splint	0	1	4.0 × 24 in	10.2 × 61 cm
Sterile pad	2	4	3 × 3 in	7.5 × 7.5 cm
Tourniquet	0	1	1 in (width)	2.5 cm (width)
Trauma pad	2	4	5 × 9 in	12.7 × 22.9 cm
Triangular bandage	1	2	40 × 40 × 56 in	101 × 101 × 142 cm
Directions for requesting emergency assistance (including a list of important local emergency telephone numbers, such as the police, fire department, EMS, and poison control center*)	1	1	N/A	N/A
Heartsaver First Aid CPR AED Reference Guide*	1	1	N/A	N/A

*Items marked with an asterisk are in addition to those listed in the ANSI guidelines.

Actions to Take: Maintain the First Aid Kit

- Keep the supplies in a sturdy, watertight container that is clearly labeled.
- Know where the first aid kit is.
- Replace what you use so that the kit will be ready for the next emergency.
- Check the kit at the beginning of each work period for expired supplies, and make sure it is complete and ready for an emergency.

Personal Safety

For every emergency, you will want to take these actions to protect yourself and the victim:

1. Assess the scene.
2. Take universal precautions.

Assess the Scene

First, make sure the scene is safe. Be aware of any danger for you, the ill or injured person, and anyone else nearby. Do this every time you are providing first aid or CPR. Continue to be mindful of the scene while you provide first aid or CPR for changes that could make the scene unsafe. You can't help if you're injured yourself.

Watch for Unsafe Places

Some places that may be unsafe are

- A busy street or parking lot
- An area where power lines are down
- A room with noticeable fumes

Actions to Take: Assess the Scene

When you look around, ask yourself these questions:

- Danger: Is there danger for you or the ill or injured person? Move an injured person only if they are in danger or if you need to move them to safely provide first aid or CPR.
- Help: Are others around to help? If so, have someone phone 9-1-1. If no one else is near, phone for help yourself.
- Who: Who is ill or injured? Can you tell how many people are hurt and what happened?
- Where: Where are you? You'll need to tell others how to get to you—in particular, the 9-1-1 dispatcher. If other bystanders are at the scene, send one to meet the emergency responders and lead them to the scene.

Moving an Ill or Injured Person

When giving first aid, you might wonder, "Should I move an ill or injured person?"

The answer is generally no—especially if you suspect a pelvic or spinal injury.

However, there are times when you should move the person, such as the following:

- If the area is unsafe for you or the ill or injured person, move to a safe location.
- If a person is unresponsive and breathing normally, you can roll the person onto their side. This may help keep their airway open in case they vomit.

One way to move someone is to drag them by their clothes (Figure 4). Simply grab the person's clothes at the shoulders and pull them to safety.

Figure 4. The shoulder pull is a way to move an ill or injured person.

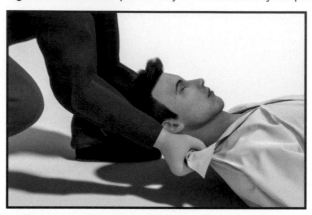

Take Universal Precautions

After you assess scene safety, there are certain precautions you should always take. These precautions are called *universal* because you should use them in every emergency. You'll use these precautions because you could come into contact with blood and other body fluids—and you should treat these fluids as though they contain germs that can cause diseases.

Personal Protective Equipment

Your first aid kit includes PPE, such as eye protection and medical gloves. Always wear them when you are giving first aid. They help keep you safe from body fluids, such as blood, saliva, and urine. The first aid kit also contains a mask for giving breaths in case you need to give CPR.

Some people are allergic to latex. Others have developed a sensitivity to latex that can cause serious reactions. This is why you should use nonlatex gloves if possible.

Actions to Take: Universal Precautions
- Wear PPE whenever necessary (Figure 5).
  - Wear protective gloves whenever you give first aid.
  - Wear eye protection if the ill or injured person is bleeding or vomiting.
- Place all disposable equipment that has touched blood or body fluids in a biohazard waste bag (Figure 6) or as required by your workplace.
  - To dispose of the biohazard waste bag, follow your company's plan for hazardous waste.
- After properly removing your gloves, wash your hands well with soap and lots of water for 20 seconds.

Figure 5. Wear protective gloves whenever you give first aid, and wear eye protection if the ill or injured person is bleeding or vomiting.

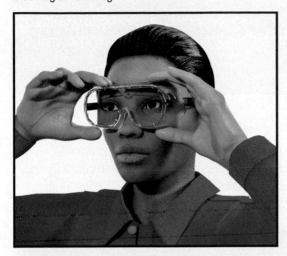

Figure 6. Place all disposable equipment that has touched body fluids, including the gloves you wore, in a biohazard waste bag if one is available. Dispose of the bag according to company policy.

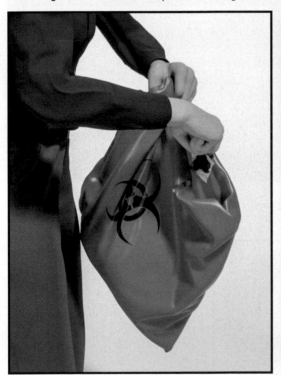
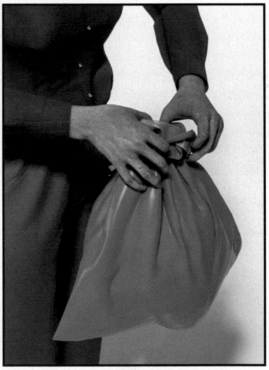

While the AHA always recommends the use of PPE and this course will often show PPE being used, it's possible you may find yourself in an emergency where PPE is unavailable. In this situation, use your best judgment for how to render first aid. If the person's blood does touch your skin or splash in your eyes or mouth, take action.

Actions to Take: Exposure to Blood

- Remove your gloves, if you are wearing them.
- Immediately wash your hands and rinse the contact area with soap and lots of water for 20 seconds.
- Rinse your eyes, your nose, or the inside of your mouth with plenty of water if body fluids splattered in any of these areas.
- Contact a healthcare provider as soon as possible.

Remove Protective Gloves Properly

Most of us have worn some type of glove in our lifetime, and you probably removed them without much thought. However, because of the risk of infection, using protective gloves and taking them off correctly are important safety steps. Always dispose of protective gloves properly so that anyone else who comes into contact with the biohazard waste bag will not be exposed to blood or other body fluids.

Actions to Take: Remove Protective Gloves

- Grip one glove on the outside near the cuff and peel it down until it comes off inside out (Figure 7A).
- Cup it with your other gloved hand (Figure 7B).
- Place 2 fingers of your bare hand inside the cuff of the glove that is still on your other hand (Figure 7C).
- Peel that glove off so that it comes off inside out with the first glove inside of it (Figure 7D).
- If blood or blood-containing material is on the gloves, dispose of the gloves properly.
  - Put the gloves in a biohazard waste bag.
  - If you do not have a biohazard waste bag, put the gloves in a plastic bag that can be sealed before you dispose of it.
- Always wash your hands after removing gloves, just in case blood or other body fluids came into contact with your hands.

Figure 7. Proper removal of protective gloves without touching the outside of the gloves.

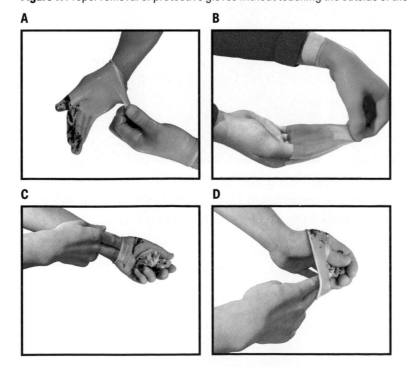

A B

C D

Practice Good Hand Hygiene

Even if you've been wearing protective gloves, wash your hands in case body fluids came into contact with them. Washing your hands often and not touching your face is one of the best things you can do for your health and the health of those around you, even if you haven't been exposed to blood or other body fluids.

Actions to Take: Wash Hands Well

- Wet your hands with clean running water (warm if available) and apply soap.
- Rub hands together and scrub all surfaces of hands and fingers for at least 20 seconds (Figure 8).
- Rinse hands with lots of running water.
- Dry your hands using a paper towel or air dryer. If possible, use your paper towel to turn off the faucet.

Figure 8. Wash your hands well with soap and lots of water after taking off your gloves.

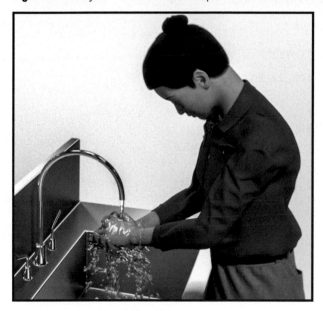

Using Waterless Hand Sanitizer

If you can't wash your hands right away, use waterless hand sanitizer. Rub your hands together so that the sanitizer covers the tops and bottoms of both hands and all fingers. Then, let the sanitizer air dry.

As soon as you can, wash your hands with soap and water.

Personal Safety: Review Questions

1. When you are providing first aid, you should
   a. Wear PPE
   b. Only wear PPE if you do not know the person
   c. Not be concerned about PPE if you wash your hands
   d. Use cloth gloves to protect your hands

2. When you phone for help, you should stay on the line with the dispatcher until
   a. People with more advanced training arrive
   b. The dispatcher tells you it's OK to hang up

3. After giving first aid at your workplace, you
   a. Can talk about what happened with anyone you want
   b. Cannot discuss anything with coworkers; you must keep private things private
   c. Can speak to a reporter about the incident
   d. Can discuss the incident with your immediate coworkers only

4. You should wash your hands for at least
   a. 10 seconds
   b. 15 seconds
   c. 20 seconds
   d. 3 minutes

5. When assessing the scene, you should consider which of the following?
   a. Danger to yourself and others
   b. How many people are injured or ill
   c. Where the nearest telephone is
   d. All of the above

6. You should replace any supplies you use from the first aid kit.
   a. True
   b. False

7. Why should you wear personal protective equipment?
   a. To protect yourself from bloodborne diseases
   b. To impress people during treatment
   c. To avoid getting your own clothes dirty

8. When you provide care to an injured person at work, be sure to
   a. Write a report of the incident if your company requires it
   b. Post a report to the company bulletin board
   c. Tell the person to get a doctor's note before returning to work

9. It is important to properly remove your gloves after giving first aid so that
   a. Contaminants on the gloves can be analyzed later
   b. You don't touch the body fluids of the person you are helping
   c. The body fluids on the gloves don't touch the person you are helping

10. If you find someone unresponsive on the ground, first look for
    a. The person's cell phone
    b. The person's driver's license
    c. Medical information jewelry

Answers: 1.a, 2.b, 3.b, 4.c, 5.d, 6.a, 7.a, 8.a, 9.b, 10.c

Although much is being done to prevent death from heart problems, cardiac arrest is still a leading cause of death in the United States. And about 70% of the arrests that occur outside of the hospital happen at home. You will learn skills that will help you recognize cardiac arrest, get emergency care on the way quickly, and help the person until more advanced care arrives to take over.

In this section, you will learn when CPR is needed, how to give CPR to an adult, and how to use an AED.

Adult Chain of Survival

The AHA adult Chain of Survival (Figure 9) shows the most important actions needed to treat adults who have cardiac arrests outside of a hospital. During this course, you will learn about the first 3 links of the chain. The fourth and fifth links are advanced care provided by emergency responders and hospital providers who take over care, and the sixth link is recovery.

Remember that seconds count when someone has a cardiac arrest. Wherever you are, take action. The adult Chain of Survival starts with you!

- **First link:** Immediately recognize the emergency and phone 9-1-1.
- **Second link:** Perform early CPR with an emphasis on chest compressions.
- **Third link:** Use an AED immediately (as soon as it is available).
- **Fourth and fifth links:** Advanced care is provided.
- **Sixth link:** Additional treatment, observation, and rehabilitation may be needed to fully recover from a cardiac arrest.

Figure 9. The AHA adult Chain of Survival for cardiac arrests that occur outside of a hospital.

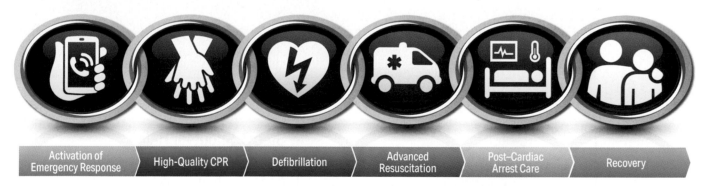

| Activation of Emergency Response | High-Quality CPR | Defibrillation | Advanced Resuscitation | Post-Cardiac Arrest Care | Recovery |

Assess and Phone 9-1-1

When you see an adult who may have had a cardiac arrest, take the following 5 steps to assess the emergency and get help.

1. Make sure the scene is safe.
2. Tap and shout (check for responsiveness).
3. Shout for help.
4. Phone 9-1-1 and get an AED.
5. Check for normal breathing.

Depending on the circumstance and the resources you have available, you may be able to take some of these actions at the same time. You might, for example, phone 9-1-1 with your cell phone on speaker mode while you are checking for breathing.

The following details about each of these steps will help you assess a medical emergency.

Step 1: Make Sure the Scene Is Safe

Before you begin to help the person, look for anything nearby that might hurt you. You can't help if you get hurt too.

As you help, be aware if anything changes and makes it unsafe for you or the person.

Step 2: Tap and Shout (Check for Responsiveness)

Actions to Take: Check for Responsiveness
- Tap their shoulders and shout to check whether the person is responsive or unresponsive (Figure 10).
- If the person is responsive, ask if they need help.
- If the person is unresponsive, shout for help so that if others are nearby, they can help you.

Figure 10. Tap and shout (check for responsiveness).

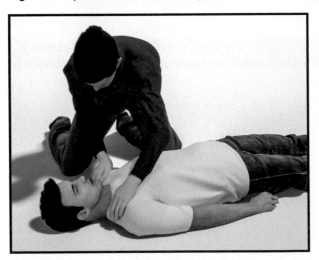

Step 3: Shout for Help

In an emergency, the sooner you realize that there's a problem and get help, the better it is for the person with a cardiac arrest. When more people are helping, you can provide better care.

If the person you are helping is unresponsive, shout for help (Figure 11).

Figure 11. Shout for help.

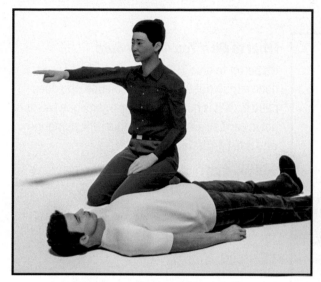

Step 4: Phone 9-1-1 and Get an AED

If someone comes to help and a cell phone is available

Ask the person to phone 9-1-1 and get an AED. Say, "You—phone 9-1-1 and get an AED." Ask the person to put the phone on speaker mode so that you can hear the dispatcher's instructions.

If someone comes to help and a cell phone is not available

Ask the person to go phone 9-1-1 and get an AED while you continue providing emergency care.

If you are alone and have a cell phone or nearby phone

If no one comes to help, phone 9-1-1. Put the phone on speaker mode so that you can hear the dispatcher's instructions while you provide emergency care. If you need an AED, you will have to go get it yourself.

If you are alone and don't have a cell phone

Leave the person while you go to phone 9-1-1 and get an AED. Return and continue providing emergency care.

Follow the Dispatcher's Instructions

Stay on the phone until the 9-1-1 dispatcher tells you to hang up. Answering the dispatcher's questions will not delay the arrival of help.

The dispatcher will ask you about the emergency—where you are and what has happened. Dispatchers can provide instructions that will help you, such as telling you how to provide CPR, use an AED, or give first aid.

That's why it's important to put the phone on speaker mode after phoning 9-1-1. It allows the dispatcher and the person providing CPR to speak to each other.

Step 5: Check for Breathing

If the person is unresponsive, check for breathing (Figure 12). Scan the chest repeatedly for at least 5 seconds (but no more than 10 seconds), looking for the chest to rise and fall. If the person is not breathing normally or is only gasping, they need CPR.

Actions to Take: Check for Breathing

If the person is unresponsive and is breathing

- This person does not need CPR.
- Roll them onto their side (if you don't suspect a neck or back injury). This will help keep the airway clear in case the person vomits.
- Stay with the person until advanced help arrives.

If the person is unresponsive and not breathing or is only gasping

- This person needs CPR.
- Make sure the person is lying faceup on a firm, flat surface.
- Begin CPR.

Remember: Unresponsive + No breathing or only gasping = Provide CPR

Figure 12. Check for breathing.

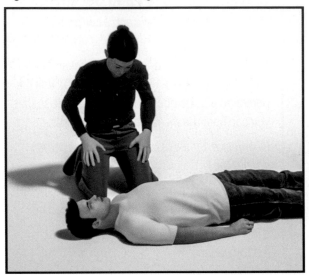

What to Do if You Are Not Sure

It's better to give CPR to someone who doesn't need it than not to give it to someone who does need it. CPR is not likely to harm someone who is not in cardiac arrest. But without CPR, someone who is in cardiac arrest may die.

So if you aren't sure, provide CPR. You may save a life.

Summary

Here is a summary of how to assess the emergency and get help when you encounter an ill or injured adult:

Assess and Phone 9-1-1
- Make sure the scene is safe.
- Tap and shout (check for responsiveness).
  - If the person is responsive, ask, "Do you need help?"
  - If the person is unresponsive, go to the next step.
- Shout for help.
- Phone 9-1-1 and get an AED.
  - Phone or send someone else to phone 9-1-1 and get an AED.
  - If you're alone and have a cell phone or a nearby phone, put it on speaker mode and phone 9-1-1.
  - If you're alone and don't have a nearby phone, leave the person while you go phone 9-1-1 and get an AED.
- Check for breathing.
  - If the person is breathing normally, stay with the person until advanced help arrives.
  - If the person is not breathing normally or is only gasping, begin CPR and use an AED.

Perform High-Quality CPR

Learning how to perform high-quality CPR is important. The better you can perform CPR skills, the better the chances of survival, whether you are helping an adult, a child, or an infant.

CPR has 2 main skills:

- Providing compressions
- Giving breaths

In this section, you will learn how to perform these skills for an adult in cardiac arrest. The AHA encourages bystanders who are not trained in CPR to give compression-only CPR, or Hands-Only CPR, if they see a teen or an adult collapse. In the first few minutes of cardiac arrest, survival rates of those who have received Hands-Only CPR and those who have received CPR with breaths are similar. There are 2 simple steps to follow: phone 9-1-1, and push hard and fast in the center of the chest. If you are willing and able to give breaths, you should do so, especially for children or anyone who might be in cardiac arrest due to respiratory issues such as drowning or drug overdose.

Provide Compressions

To provide high-quality compressions, make sure that you

- Provide compressions that are deep enough
- Provide compressions that are fast enough
- Let the chest come back up to its normal position after each compression
- Try not to interrupt compressions for more than 10 seconds, even when you give breaths

Compression depth is an important part of providing high-quality compressions. You need to push hard enough to pump blood through the body. It's better to push too hard than not hard enough. People are often afraid of injuring a person by providing compressions, but injury is unlikely.

Actions to Take: Provide Compressions for an Adult

- Make sure the person is lying faceup on a firm, flat surface.
- Quickly move bulky clothes out of the way. If a person's clothes are difficult to remove, you can still provide compressions over clothing.
  - If an AED becomes available, remove all clothes that cover the chest. AED pads must not be placed over any clothing.
- Put the heel of one hand on the center of the person's chest, over the lower half of the breastbone (Figure 13A). Put your other hand on top of the first hand (Figure 13B).
- Push straight down at least 2 inches, or 5 cm.
- Push at a rate of 100 to 120/min. Count the compressions out loud.
- Let the chest come back up to its normal position after each compression.
- Try not to interrupt chest compressions for more than 10 seconds, even when you give breaths.

Compressions for a Pregnant Woman

- Do not delay providing chest compressions for a pregnant woman in cardiac arrest. High-quality CPR can increase the mother's and the infant's chance of survival. If you do not perform CPR on a pregnant woman when needed, the lives of both the mother and the infant are at risk.
- Perform high-quality chest compressions for a pregnant woman in cardiac arrest the same way you would for any victim of cardiac arrest. If the woman begins to move, speak, blink, or otherwise react, stop CPR and roll her onto her left side.

Figure 13. Compressions. **A,** Put the heel of one hand on the center of the chest (lower half of the breastbone). **B,** Put the other hand on top of the first hand.

A

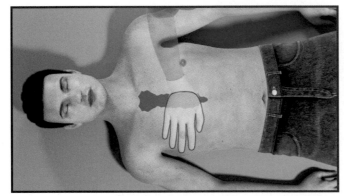

B

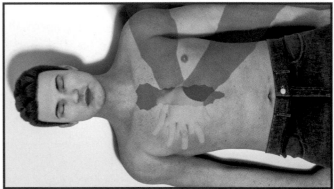

Switch Rescuers to Avoid Fatigue

Performing chest compressions correctly is hard work. The more tired you become, the less effective your compressions will be.

If someone else knows CPR, you can take turns providing compressions (Figure 14). Switch rescuers about every 2 minutes, or sooner if you get tired. Move quickly to keep any pauses in compressions as short as possible.

Remind other rescuers to perform high-quality CPR as described in the box Actions to Take: Provide Compressions for an Adult.

Figure 14. Switch rescuers about every 2 minutes to avoid fatigue.

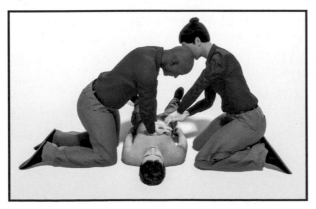

Give Breaths

The second skill of CPR is giving breaths. After each set of 30 compressions, you will need to give 2 breaths.

When you give breaths, the breaths need to make the chest rise visibly. When you can see the chest rise, you know you have given an effective breath.

Open the Airway

Before giving breaths, open the airway (Figure 15). This lifts the tongue from the back of the throat to make sure your breaths get air into the lungs.

Actions to Take: Open the Airway

- Put one hand on the forehead and the fingers of your other hand on the bony part of the chin (Figure 15). Avoid pressing into the soft part of the neck or under the chin because this might block the airway.
- Tilt the head back and lift the chin.

Figure 15. Open the airway by tilting the head back and lifting the chin.

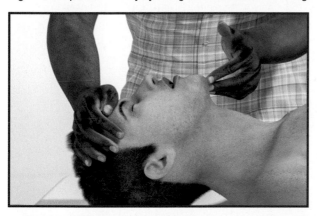

Give Sets of 30 Compressions and 2 Breaths

When providing CPR, give sets of 30 compressions and 2 breaths.

Give Breaths Without a Pocket Mask

Giving someone breaths without a barrier device is usually quite safe. Use your best judgment on whether it is safe for you to give breaths.

Actions to Take: Give Breaths Without a Pocket Mask

- While holding the airway open, pinch the nose closed with your thumb and forefinger.
- Take a normal breath. Cover the person's mouth with your mouth (Figure 16).
- Give 2 breaths (blow for 1 second for each). Watch for the chest to begin to rise as you give each breath.
- Try not to interrupt chest compressions for more than 10 seconds, even when you give breaths.

Figure 16. Giving breaths without a barrier device.

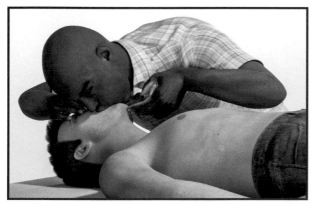

Pocket Masks for Giving Breaths

You can give breaths with or without a barrier device, such as a pocket mask. These plastic devices fit over the person's mouth and nose (Figure 17). They protect the rescuer from blood, vomit, or disease. Your instructor may discuss other types of barrier devices, like face shields, that you can use when giving breaths.

If you're in the workplace, your employer may provide PPE that includes pocket masks or face shields to use during CPR.

There are different kinds of pocket masks as well as different sizes for adults, children, and infants. So make sure you're using the right size. Pocket masks are typically made of hard plastic with a 1-way valve, which is the part you breathe into. You may need to put a pocket mask together before you use it. To put it together, push the plastic dome into place by using your thumbs to pop it out. Then, attach the 1-way valve.

Figure 17. Some people use a pocket mask when giving breaths.

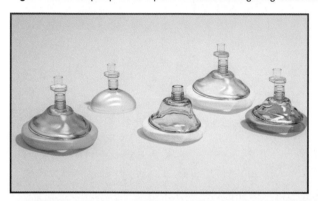

Give Breaths With a Pocket Mask

As you give each breath, look at the person's chest to see if it begins to rise. Seeing the chest begin to rise is the best way to know that your breaths are effective.

Actions to Take: Give Breaths With a Pocket Mask

- Put the mask over the person's mouth and nose.
  - If the mask has a narrow, pointed end, put that end on the bridge of the nose; position the wide end so that it covers the mouth.
- Tilt the head and lift the chin while pressing the mask against the person's face (Figure 18). It is important to make an airtight seal between the person's face and the mask while you lift the chin to keep the airway open.
- Give 2 breaths (blow for 1 second for each). Watch for the chest to begin to rise as you give each breath.
- Try not to interrupt chest compressions for more than 10 seconds, even when you give breaths.

Figure 18. Giving breaths with a pocket mask.

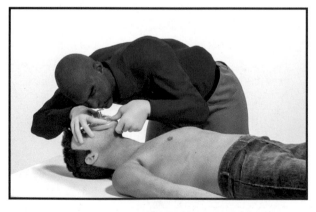

What to Do if the Chest Doesn't Rise

It takes a little practice to give breaths correctly. If you give someone a breath and the chest doesn't rise, do the following:

- Allow the head to go back to its normal position.
- Open the airway again by tilting the head back and lifting the chin.
- Then, give another breath. Make sure the chest rises.

Minimize Interruptions in Chest Compressions

If you have been unable to give 2 effective breaths in 10 seconds, go back to pushing hard and fast on the chest. Try to give breaths again after every 30 compressions. Don't interrupt compressions for more than 10 seconds.

Actions to Take: Provide Adult CPR

- Make sure the person is lying faceup on a firm, flat surface.
- Quickly move bulky clothes out of the way. If a person's clothes are difficult to remove, you can still provide compressions over clothing.
  - If an AED becomes available, remove all clothes that cover the chest. AED pads must not be placed over any clothing.
- Give 30 chest compressions.
  - Put the heel of one hand on the center of the chest (over the lower half of the breastbone). Put your other hand on top of the first hand.
  - Push straight down at least 2 inches.
  - Push at a rate of 100 to 120/min. Count the compressions out loud.
  - Let the chest come back up to its normal position after each compression.
- After 30 compressions, give 2 breaths.
  - Open the airway and give 2 breaths (blow for 1 second for each). Watch for the chest to begin to rise as you give each breath.
- Try not to interrupt compressions for more than 10 seconds, even when you give breaths.

Use an AED

CPR combined with using an AED provides the best chance of saving a life. If possible, use an AED every time you provide CPR.

AEDs are safe, accurate, and easy to use. Once you turn on the AED, follow the prompts. The AED will check to see if the person needs a shock and will automatically give one or tell you when to give one.

AED Pads

AEDs may have 2 sets of pads: adult pads and child pads. For CPR, you learned that a child is anyone 1 year or older who has not gone through puberty. However, for defibrillation, make sure you use the adult pads for anyone 8 years or older. Before you place the pads, quickly scan the person to check for special situations that might require additional steps. See Special Situations later in this section.

Actions to Take: Use an AED for an Adult

- Turn the AED on and follow the prompts.
  - Turn it on by pushing the On button or lifting the lid (Figure 19).
  - Follow the prompts, which will tell you everything you need to do.
- Attach the adult pads.
  - Use the adult pads for anyone 8 years or older.
  - Peel away the backing from the pads.
  - Following the pictures on the pads, attach them to the person's bare chest (Figure 20).
  - Plug the pads connector into the AED, if necessary.

(continued)

Actions to Take: Use an AED for an Adult *(continued)*

- Let the AED analyze.
  - Loudly state, "Clear," and make sure that no one is touching the person.
  - The AED will analyze the heart rhythm.
  - If the AED tells you that a shock is not needed, resume CPR.
- Deliver a shock if needed (Figure 21).
  - Loudly state, "Clear," and make sure that no one is touching the person.
  - Push the Shock button.
- Immediately resume CPR.

Figure 19. Turn on the AED.

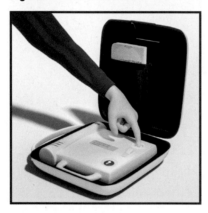

Figure 20. Place pads on an adult by following the pictures on the pads.

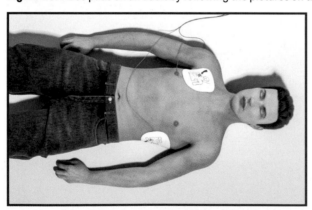

Figure 21. Make sure that no one is touching the person just before you push the Shock button.

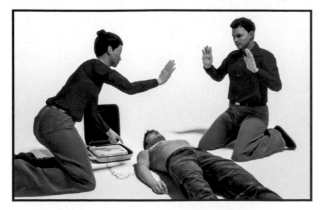

Special Situations

Some special situations can affect how you should place the AED pads. So before you apply the pads, quickly scan the person and assess the situation to check for the following:

Actions to Take: Special Situations

Hairy Chest

If the person has hair on the chest that may prevent pads from sticking, remove the hair in one of these ways:

- Quickly shave the area where you will place the pads by using the razor from the AED carrying case (Figure 22).
- Use a second set of AED pads (if available) to remove the hair (Figure 23).
  - Apply the pads and press them down firmly.
  - Rip the pads off forcefully to remove the chest hair.
  - Reapply a new set of pads to the bare skin.

Water on or Near Person

If the person is lying in water

- Quickly move the person to a dry area.

If the person is lying on snow or in a small puddle

- You can use the AED (the chest doesn't have to be completely dry).
- If the chest is covered with water or sweat, quickly wipe it before attaching the pads.

If there is water on the person's chest

- Quickly wipe the chest dry before attaching the pads (Figure 24).

Implanted Pacemaker

If the person has an implanted defibrillator or pacemaker

- Don't put the AED pad directly over the implanted device (Figure 25).
- Follow the normal steps for operating an AED.

Medicine Patch

If there is a medicine patch where you need to place an AED pad

- Don't put the AED pad directly over a medicine patch (Figure 26).
- Use protective gloves.
- Remove the medicated patch.
- Wipe the area clean.
- Attach the AED pads.

Jewelry or Bra/Undergarment

- You don't need to remove a person's jewelry as long as it does not interfere with the placement of the pads and is not in contact with the pads. It does not cause a shock hazard to either the person or rescuer.
- Undergarments should be removed, along with other clothes covering the chest, because they often interfere with proper pad placement.

(continued)

Figure 22. If the AED contains a razor, use it to shave a hairy chest.

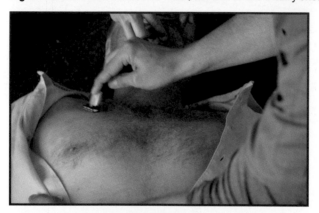

Figure 23. If the AED contains 2 sets of pads, use 1 set to remove the hair on a hairy chest.

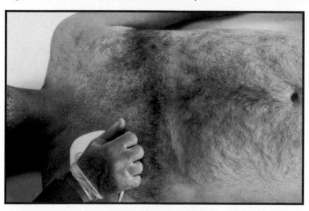

Figure 24. Wipe excess water off the chest.

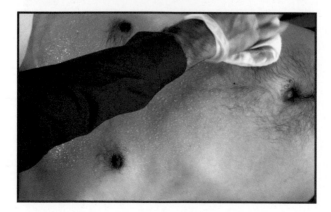

Figure 25. Don't apply AED pad over implanted device.

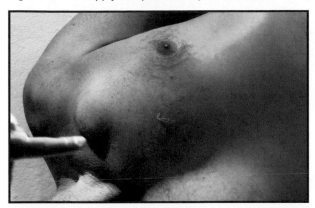

Figure 26. Don't apply AED pad over medicine patch.

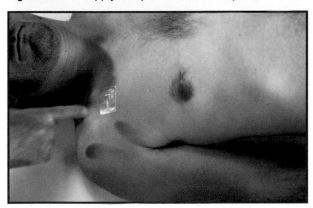

Continue Providing CPR and Using the AED

As soon as the AED gives the shock, immediately resume chest compressions. Continue to follow the AED prompts, which will guide you.

Provide CPR and use the AED until

- Someone else arrives who can take turns providing CPR with you
  - If someone else arrives, you can take turns giving compressions. Switch rescuers about every 2 minutes, which is about 5 cycles of compressions or breaths, or sooner if you get tired.
- The person begins to move, speak, blink, or otherwise react
- Someone with more advanced training arrives

Putting It All Together:
Adult High-Quality CPR AED Summary

Compressions are very important to deliver blood flow. They are the core of CPR. Try not to interrupt chest compressions for more than 10 seconds when you give breaths.

Assess and Phone 9-1-1
- Make sure the scene is safe.
- Tap and shout (check for responsiveness).
  - If the person is responsive, ask, "Do you need help?"
  - If the person is unresponsive, go to the next step.
- Shout for help.
- Phone 9-1-1 and get an AED.
  - Phone or send someone else to phone 9-1-1 and get an AED.
  - If you're alone and have a cell phone or nearby phone, put it on speaker mode and phone 9-1-1.
  - If you're alone and don't have a nearby phone, leave the person while you go phone 9-1-1 and get an AED.
- Check for breathing.
  - If the person is breathing, stay with the person until advanced help arrives.
  - If the person is not breathing or is only gasping, begin CPR and use the AED. See the next steps.

Provide High-Quality CPR
When providing CPR, give sets of 30 compressions and 2 breaths.

- Make sure the person is lying faceup on a firm, flat surface.
- Quickly move bulky clothes out of the way. If a person's clothes are difficult to remove, you can still provide compressions over clothing.
  - If an AED becomes available, remove all clothes that cover the chest. AED pads must not be placed over any clothing.
- Give 30 chest compressions.
  - Put the heel of one hand on the center of the chest (over the lower half of the breastbone). Put your other hand on top of the first hand.
  - Push straight down at least 2 inches, or 5 cm.
  - Push at a rate of 100 to 120/min. Count the compressions out loud.
  - Let the chest come back up to its normal position after each compression.
- After 30 compressions, give 2 breaths.
  - Open the airway and give 2 breaths (blow for 1 second for each). As you give each breath, watch for the chest to begin to rise.
  - Try not to interrupt compressions for more than 10 seconds, even when you give breaths.
- Use an AED as soon as it is available.
  - Turn the AED on and follow the prompts.
  - Attach the adult pads.
  - Let the AED analyze.
  - Make sure that no one is touching the person, and deliver a shock if advised.
- Provide CPR and use the AED until
  - Someone else arrives who can take turns providing CPR with you
  - The person begins to move, speak, blink, or otherwise react
  - Someone with more advanced training arrives and takes over

Drug Overdose Emergency

How to Help an Adult With a Drug Overdose Emergency

Across the world, far too many people are dying from drug overdoses. These deaths are largely due to opioids. Common opioids are morphine, fentanyl, heroin, oxycodone, methadone, and hydrocodone.

Naloxone is a medication used to reverse the overdose effects of an opioid and help the person to survive. It is safe and effective. Emergency responders have used naloxone for many years.

Family members or caregivers of known opioid users may keep naloxone close by to use in case of an opioid overdose. An accidental overdose can happen to anyone. If you know someone who has access to naloxone, you may need to use it. It is important to be familiar with how to use naloxone.

Facts About Naloxone

- Naloxone is available without a prescription in most states and through substance use disorder treatment programs.
- Naloxone comes in several forms. Common forms are an intranasal spray and an autoinjector (similar to an epinephrine pen).
- Give naloxone by spraying it into the nose or by injecting it with an autoinjector into a muscle.
- Naloxone is used only to reverse the effects of an opioid overdose. It won't work for other types of drug overdoses.

Opioid-Associated Emergency

Common signs of opioid overdose include unresponsiveness with shallow or slow breathing, or even no breathing or only gasping. You may suspect a drug overdose if you see signs of drugs nearby or if there's other evidence of drug use. If you suspect that someone has had an opioid overdose and the person is still responsive, phone 9-1-1 and stay with the person until someone with more advanced training arrives.

Actions to Take: Help an Adult With an Opioid-Associated Emergency

- Make sure the scene is safe.
- Tap and shout (check for responsiveness).
- Shout for help.
- Phone 9-1-1 and get the naloxone kit and an AED.
  - Phone or send someone else to phone 9-1-1 and get the naloxone kit and an AED.
  - If you're alone and have a cell phone or nearby phone, put it on speaker mode and phone 9-1-1.
- Check for breathing.
  - If the person is breathing normally, give naloxone if available, and stay with the person until advanced help arrives.
  - If the person is not breathing normally or is only gasping, provide CPR, and use the AED as soon as it is available. Give the naloxone as soon as you can, but do not delay CPR to give naloxone.
- Continue giving CPR and using the AED until
  - Someone else arrives who can take turns providing CPR with you
  - The person begins to move, speak, blink, or otherwise react
  - Someone with more advanced training arrives

CPR and AED Use for Children

If you are not sure whether someone is an adult or a child, provide emergency care as if the person is an adult. But note that the definition of *child* is different when using an AED compared with providing CPR. See Use an AED later in this section.

Pediatric Chain of Survival

The AHA pediatric Chain of Survival (Figure 27) shows the most important actions needed to treat children who have cardiac arrests outside of a hospital. During this course, you will learn about the first 3 links of the chain. The fourth and fifth links are advanced care provided by emergency responders and hospital providers who will take over care, and the sixth link is recovery.

Remember that seconds count when a child has a cardiac arrest. Wherever you are, take action. The pediatric Chain of Survival starts with you!

- **First link:** Preventing injury and cardiac arrest is an important first step in saving children's lives.
- **Second link:** Phoning 9-1-1 as soon as possible so that the child can have emergency care quickly improves outcome.
- **Third link:** The sooner that high-quality CPR is started for someone in cardiac arrest, the better the chances of survival.
- **Fourth and fifth links:** Advanced care is provided.
- **Sixth link:** A child may need continued care and support for months or years to fully recover after a cardiac arrest.

Figure 27. The AHA pediatric Chain of Survival for cardiac arrests that occur outside of a hospital.

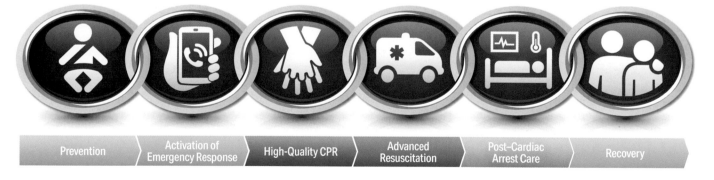

| Prevention | Activation of Emergency Response | High-Quality CPR | Advanced Resuscitation | Post–Cardiac Arrest Care | Recovery |

Cardiac Arrest in Children

Children usually have healthy hearts, but they can have respiratory problems that cause them to need CPR. Other emergencies that can lead to cardiac arrest in children are drowning, trauma, and electrical injury. In the pediatric Chain of Survival, preventing cardiac arrest is one of the most important things you can do. This includes the prevention of drowning, choking, and other respiratory problems.

Because respiratory problems are often the cause of cardiac arrest in children, if a child is in cardiac arrest and you are alone and do not have a phone nearby, you will provide CPR for 2 minutes (5 sets of compressions and breaths) before leaving to phone 9-1-1.

Assess and Phone 9-1-1

When you see a child who may have had a cardiac arrest, take the following 5 steps to assess the emergency and get help:

1. Make sure the scene is safe.
2. Tap and shout (check for responsiveness).
3. Shout for help.
4. Check for breathing.
5. Phone 9-1-1, begin CPR, and get an AED.

Depending on the circumstance and the resources you have available, you may be able to perform some of these actions at the same time. You might, for example, phone 9-1-1 with your cell phone on speaker mode while checking for breathing.

The following details about each of these steps will help you assess a medical emergency.

Step 1: Make Sure the Scene Is Safe

Before you begin to help the child, look for anything nearby that might hurt you. You can't help if you get hurt too.

As you help, be aware if anything changes and makes it unsafe for you or the child.

Step 2: Tap and Shout (Check for Responsiveness)

Actions to Take: Check for Responsiveness
- Tap their shoulders and shout to check whether the child is responsive or unresponsive (Figure 28).
    - If the child is responsive, ask if they need help.
    - If the child is unresponsive, shout for help so that if others are nearby, they can help you.

Figure 28. Tap and shout (check for responsiveness).

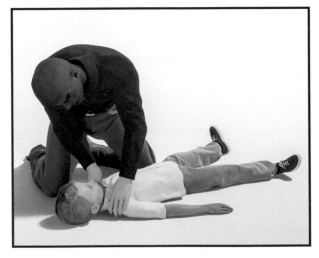

Step 3: Shout for Help

In an emergency, the sooner you realize that there's a problem and get help, the better it is for the child with a cardiac arrest. When more people are helping, you can provide better care.

If the child is unresponsive, shout for help (Figure 29). If someone comes, send that person to phone 9-1-1 and get an AED. If you have a cell phone, phone 9-1-1 and put it on speaker mode.

Figure 29. Shout for help.

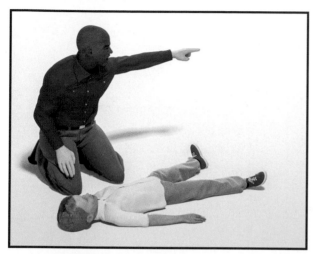

Step 4: Check for Breathing

If the child is unresponsive, check for breathing (Figure 30). Scan the chest repeatedly for at least 5 seconds (but no more than 10 seconds), looking for the chest to rise and fall. If the child is not breathing or is only gasping, they need CPR.

Actions to Take: Check for Breathing

If the child is unresponsive and is breathing

- This child does not need CPR.
- Roll them onto their side (if you don't suspect a neck or back injury). This will help keep the airway clear in case the child vomits.
- Stay with the child until advanced help arrives.

If the child is unresponsive and is not breathing or is only gasping

- This child needs CPR.
- Make sure the child is lying faceup on a firm, flat surface.
- Have someone phone 9-1-1, or use your cell phone (or nearby phone), put it on speaker mode, and phone 9-1-1.
- Begin CPR. Give 5 sets of 30 compressions and 2 breaths.
- After 5 sets of compressions and breaths, phone 9-1-1 and get an AED (if no one has done this yet). Use the AED as soon as it is available.
- Resume CPR and using the AED until advanced help arrives and takes over.

Remember: **Unresponsive + No breathing or only gasping = Provide CPR**

Figure 30. Check for breathing.

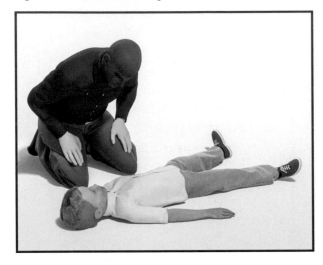

Step 5: Phone 9-1-1, Begin CPR, and Get an AED

If someone comes to help and a cell phone is available

- Ask the person to phone 9-1-1 on the cell phone, put it on speaker mode, and go get an AED while you begin CPR.
- Use the AED as soon as it is available.

If someone comes to help and a cell phone is not available

- Ask the person to go phone 9-1-1 and get an AED while you begin CPR.
- Use the AED as soon as it is available.

If you are alone and have a cell phone or a nearby phone

- Phone 9-1-1 and put the phone on speaker mode while you begin CPR.
- Give 5 sets of 30 compressions and 2 breaths.
- Go get an AED. Use it as soon as it is available.
- Return to the child and continue CPR.

If you are alone and don't have a cell phone

- Give 5 sets of 30 compressions and 2 breaths.
- Go phone 9-1-1 and get an AED. Use the AED as soon as it is available.
- Return to the child and continue CPR.
- Continue providing CPR and using the AED until
  - Someone else arrives who can take turns providing CPR with you
  - The child begins to move, speak, blink, or otherwise react
  - Someone with more advanced training arrives

Follow the Dispatcher's Instructions

Stay on the phone until the 9-1-1 dispatcher tells you to hang up. Answering the dispatcher's questions will not delay the arrival of help.

The dispatcher will ask you about the emergency—where you are and what has happened. Dispatchers can provide instructions that will help you, such as telling you how to provide CPR, use an AED, or give first aid.

That's why it's important to put the phone on speaker mode after phoning 9-1-1. It allows the dispatcher and the person providing CPR to speak to each other.

What to Do if You Are Not Sure

It's better to give CPR to a child who doesn't need it than not to give it to a child who does need it. CPR is not likely to cause harm if the child is not in cardiac arrest. But without CPR, a child who is in cardiac arrest may die.

So if you aren't sure, provide CPR. You may save a child's life.

Summary

Here is a summary of how to assess the emergency and get help when you encounter an ill or injured child:

Assess and Get Help
- Make sure the scene is safe.
- Tap and shout (check for responsiveness).
  - If the child is responsive, ask, "Do you need help?"
  - If the child is unresponsive, go to the next step.
- Shout for help.
- Check for breathing.
  - If the child is breathing, stay with the child until advanced help arrives.
  - If the child is not breathing or is only gasping, begin CPR and use an AED. See the next steps.

Phone 9-1-1, Begin CPR, and Get an AED
- Make sure the child is lying faceup on a firm, flat surface.
- Quickly move bulky clothes out of the way. If a child's clothes are difficult to remove, you can still provide compressions over clothing.
  - If an AED becomes available, remove all clothes that cover the chest. AED pads must not be placed over any clothing.

If someone comes to help and a cell phone is available

- Ask the person to phone 9-1-1 on the cell phone, put it on speaker mode, and go get an AED while you begin CPR.
- Use the AED as soon as it is available.

If someone comes to help and a cell phone is not available

- Ask the person to go phone 9-1-1 and get an AED while you begin CPR.
- Use the AED as soon as it is available.

If you are alone and have a cell phone or a nearby phone

- Phone 9-1-1 and put the phone on speaker mode while you begin CPR.
- Give 5 sets of 30 compressions and 2 breaths.
- Go get an AED, and use it as soon as it is available.
- Return to the child and continue CPR.

If you are alone and don't have a cell phone

- Give 5 sets of 30 compressions and 2 breaths.
- Go phone 9-1-1 and get an AED, and use it as soon as it is available.
- Return to the child and continue CPR.
- Continue providing CPR and using the AED until
  - Someone else arrives who can take turns providing CPR with you
  - The child begins to move, speak, blink, or otherwise react
  - Someone with more advanced training arrives

Perform High-Quality CPR

Learning how to perform high-quality CPR is important. The better you can perform CPR skills, the better the person's chances of survival, whether you are helping an adult, a child, or an infant.

CPR has 2 main skills:

- Providing compressions
- Giving breaths

In this section, you will learn how to perform these skills for a child in cardiac arrest.

Provide Compressions

To perform high-quality compressions, make sure that you

- Provide compressions that are deep enough
- Provide compressions that are fast enough
- Let the chest come back up to its normal position after each compression
- Try not to interrupt compressions for more than 10 seconds, even when you give breaths

Compression depth is an important part of providing high-quality compressions. You need to push hard enough to pump blood through the body. It's better to push too hard than not hard enough. People are often afraid of injuring a child by providing compressions, but injury is unlikely.

Compression Technique

When providing compressions for a child, use 1 hand (Figure 31). If you can't push down at least one third the depth of the child's chest (or approximately 2 inches) with 1 hand, use 2 hands to compress the chest (Figure 32).

Actions to Take: Provide Compressions for a Child

- Make sure the child is lying faceup on a firm, flat surface.
- Quickly move bulky clothes out of the way. If a child's clothes are difficult to remove, you can still provide compressions over clothing.
  - If an AED becomes available, remove all clothes that cover the chest. AED pads must not be placed over any clothing.
- Use 1 or 2 hands to give compressions.
  - **1 hand:** Put the heel of one hand on the center of the child's chest, over the lower half of the breastbone.
  - **2 hands:** Put the heel of one hand on the center of the child's chest, over the lower half of the breastbone. Put your other hand on top of the first hand.
- Push straight down at least one third the depth of the chest, or approximately 2 inches.
- Push at a rate of 100 to 120/min. Count the compressions out loud.
- Let the chest come back up to its normal position after each compression.
- **Try not to interrupt chest compressions for more than 10 seconds, even when you give breaths.**

Figure 31. Using 1 hand to give compressions to a child.

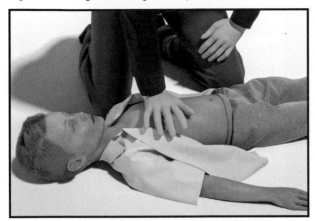

Figure 32. Using 2 hands to give compressions to a child.

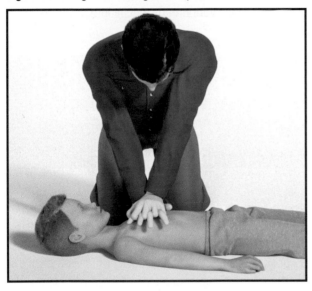

Switch Rescuers to Avoid Fatigue

Performing chest compressions correctly is hard work. The more tired you become, the less effective your compressions will be.

If someone else knows CPR, you can take turns providing compressions (Figure 33). Switch rescuers about every 2 minutes, or sooner if you get tired. Move quickly to keep any pauses in compressions as short as possible.

Remind other rescuers to perform high-quality CPR as described in the box Actions to Take: Provide Compressions for a Child.

Figure 33. Switch rescuers about every 2 minutes to avoid fatigue.

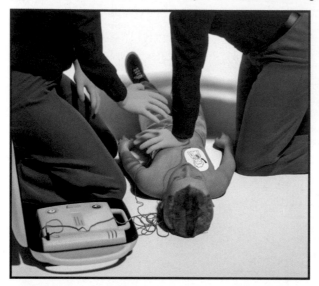

Give Breaths

The second skill of CPR is giving breaths. After each set of 30 compressions, you will need to give 2 breaths.

When you give breaths, the breaths need to make the chest rise visibly. When you can see the chest rise, you know you have delivered an effective breath.

Open the Airway

Before giving breaths, open the airway (Figure 34). This lifts the tongue from the back of the throat to make sure your breaths get air into the lungs.

Actions to Take: Open the Airway

- Put one hand on the forehead and the fingers of your other hand on the bony part of the chin (Figure 34). Avoid pressing into the soft part of the neck or under the chin because this might block the airway.
- Tilt the head back and lift the chin.

Figure 34. Open the airway by tilting the head back and lifting the chin.

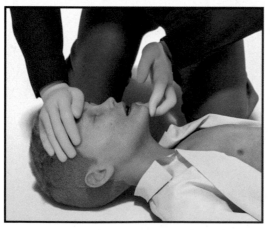

Pocket Masks for Giving Breaths

You can give breaths with or without a barrier device, such as a pocket mask. These plastic devices fit over the child's mouth and nose. They protect the rescuer from blood, vomit, or disease. Your instructor may discuss other types of barrier devices, like face shields, that you can use when giving breaths.

There are different kinds of pocket masks as well as different sizes. So make sure you're using the right size for a child. Pocket masks are typically made of hard plastic with a 1-way valve, which is the part you breathe into. You may need to put a pocket mask together before you use it.

Give Breaths Without a Pocket Mask

Giving someone breaths without a barrier device is usually quite safe. Use your best judgment on whether it is safe for you to give breaths.

Actions to Take: Give Breaths Without a Mask

- While holding the airway open, pinch the nose closed with your thumb and forefinger.
- Take a normal breath. Cover the child's mouth with your mouth (Figure 35).
- Give 2 breaths (blow for 1 second for each). Watch for the chest to begin to rise as you give each breath.
- Try not to interrupt chest compressions for more than 10 seconds, even when you give breaths.

Figure 35. Cover the child's mouth with your mouth.

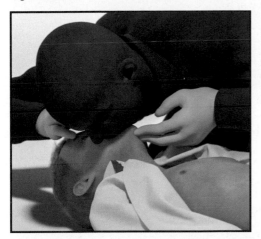

Give Breaths With a Pocket Mask

As you give each breath, look at the child's chest to see if it begins to rise. For small children, you will not need to blow as much as for larger children. Seeing the chest begin to rise is the best way to know that your breaths are effective.

Actions to Take: Give Breaths With a Pocket Mask

- Put the mask over the child's mouth and nose.
  - If the mask has a narrow, pointed end, put that end of the mask on the bridge of the nose; position the wide end so that it covers the mouth.
- Tilt the head and lift the chin while pressing the mask against the child's face. It is important to make an airtight seal between the child's face and the mask while you lift the chin to keep the airway open.
- Give 2 breaths (blow for 1 second for each). Watch for the chest to begin to rise as you give each breath (Figure 36).
- Try not to interrupt chest compressions for more than 10 seconds, even when you give breaths.

Figure 36. Giving breaths with a pocket mask.

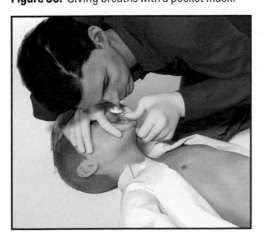

What to Do if the Chest Doesn't Rise

It takes a little practice to give breaths correctly. If you give someone a breath and the chest doesn't rise, do the following:

- Allow the head to go back to its normal position.
- Open the airway again by tilting the head back and lifting the chin.
- Then, give another breath. Make sure the chest rises.

Minimize Interruptions in Chest Compressions

If you have been unable to give 2 effective breaths in 10 seconds, go back to pushing hard and fast on the chest. Try to give breaths again after every 30 compressions. Don't interrupt compressions for more than 10 seconds.

Actions to Take: Provide Child CPR

- Make sure the child is lying faceup on a firm, flat surface.
- Quickly move bulky clothes out of the way. If a child's clothes are difficult to remove, you can still provide compressions over clothing.
  - If an AED becomes available, remove all clothes that cover the chest. AED pads must not be placed over any clothing.
- Give 30 chest compressions.
  - Use 1 or 2 hands to give compressions.
    - **1 hand:** Put the heel of one hand on the center of the chest (over the lower half of the breastbone).
    - **2 hands:** Put the heel of one hand on the center of the chest (over the lower half of the breastbone). Put your other hand on top of the first hand.
  - Push straight down at least one third the depth of the chest, or approximately 2 inches.
  - Push at a rate of 100 to 120/min. Count the compressions out loud.
  - Let the chest come back up to its normal position after each compression.
- After 30 compressions, give 2 breaths.
  - Open the airway and give 2 breaths (blow for 1 second for each). Watch for the chest to begin to rise as you give each breath.
- Try not to interrupt compressions for more than 10 seconds, even when you give breaths.

Use an AED

CPR combined with using an AED provides the best chance of saving a life. If possible, use an AED every time you provide CPR. AEDs can be used for children and infants as well as for adults.

- Some AEDs can deliver a smaller shock dose for children and infants if you use child pads or a child-cable key or switch.
- If the AED can deliver the smaller shock dose, use it for infants and children less than 8 years of age.
- If the AED cannot deliver a child shock dose, you can use the adult pads and give an adult shock dose for infants and children less than 8 years of age.
- AEDs are safe, accurate, and easy to use. Once you turn on the AED, follow the prompts. The AED will check to see if the child needs a shock and will automatically give one or tell you when to give one.

AED Pads

- AEDs may have 2 sets of pads: adult pads and child pads. For CPR, you learned that a child is anyone 1 year of age or older who has not gone through puberty. However, for defibrillation, make sure you use the adult pads for anyone 8 years or older. Before you place the pads, quickly scan the child to see if there are any special situations that might require additional steps. See Special Situations later in this section.

Actions to Take: Use an AED for a Child

- Turn the AED on and follow the prompts.
  - Turn it on by pushing the On button or lifting the lid (Figure 37).
  - Follow the prompts, which will tell you everything you need to do.
- Attach the pads.
  - Use child pads if the child is less than 8 years of age. If child pads are not available, use adult pads.
  - Use adult pads if the child is 8 years or older.
  - Peel away the backing from the pads.
  - Following the pictures on the pads, attach them to the child's bare chest (Figure 38). Make sure the pads don't touch each other. If the pads will touch, put one pad on the child's chest and the other on the child's back.
  - Plug the pads connector into the AED, if necessary.
- Let the AED analyze.
  - Loudly state, "Clear," and make sure that no one is touching the child.
  - The AED will analyze the heart rhythm.
  - If the AED tells you that a shock is not needed, resume CPR.
- Deliver a shock if needed (Figure 39).
  - Loudly state, "Clear," and make sure that no one is touching the child.
  - Push the Shock button.
  - Immediately resume CPR.

Figure 37. Turning on the AED.

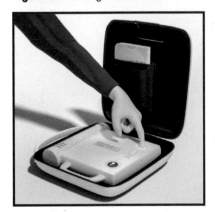

Figure 38. Place pads on a child by following the pictures on the pads.

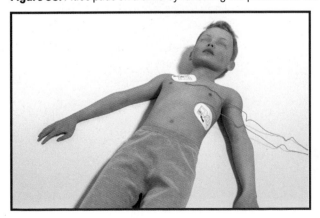

Figure 39. Make sure that no one is touching the child just before you push the Shock button.

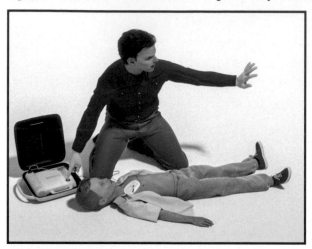

Special Situations

Some special situations can affect how you place the AED pads. Although it is not very common, you may encounter a medicine patch or a device on a child, which may interfere with the AED pad placement. So before you apply the pads, quickly scan the child and assess the situation to check for the following:

Actions to Take: Special Situations

Water on or Near Child

If the child is lying in water

- Quickly move the child to a dry area.

If the child is lying on snow or in a small puddle

- You can use the AED (the chest doesn't have to be completely dry).
- If the chest is covered with water or sweat, quickly wipe it before attaching the pads.

If there is water on the child's chest

- Quickly wipe the chest dry before attaching the pads.

Implanted Pacemaker

If the child has an implanted defibrillator or pacemaker

- Don't put the AED pad directly over the implanted device.
- Follow the normal steps for operating an AED.

Medicine Patch

If there is a medicine patch where you need to place an AED pad

- Don't put the AED pad directly over a medicine patch.
- Use protective gloves.
- Remove the medicated patch.
- Wipe the area clean.
- Attach the AED pads.

(continued)

Actions to Take: Special Situations *(continued)*

Jewelry

- You don't need to remove a child's jewelry as long as it doesn't interfere with the placement of the pads or touch the pads. It does not cause a shock hazard to either the child or rescuer.

Continue Providing CPR and Using the AED

As soon as the AED gives the shock, immediately resume chest compressions. Continue to follow the AED prompts, which will guide you.

Provide CPR and use the AED until

- Someone else arrives who can take turns providing CPR with you
  - If someone else arrives, you can take turns giving compressions. Switch rescuers about every 2 minutes, which is about 5 cycles of compressions or breaths, or sooner if you get tired.
- The child begins to move, speak, blink, or otherwise react
- Someone with more advanced training arrives

Putting It All Together: Child High-Quality CPR AED Summary

Children usually have healthy hearts. Often, a child's heart stops because the child can't breathe or is having trouble breathing. For this reason, it's very important to give breaths as well as compressions to a child.

Compressions are still very important to deliver blood flow. They are the core of CPR. Try not to interrupt chest compressions for more than 10 seconds when you give breaths.

Assess and Get Help
- Make sure the scene is safe.
- Tap and shout (check for responsiveness).
  - If the child is responsive, ask, "Do you need help?"
  - If the child is unresponsive, go to the next step.
- Shout for help.
- Check for breathing.
  - If the child is breathing, stay with the child until advanced help arrives.
  - If the child is not breathing or only gasping, begin CPR and use the AED. See the next steps.

Phone 9-1-1, Begin CPR, and Get an AED
If someone comes to help and a cell phone is available

- Ask the person to phone 9-1-1 on the cell phone, put it on speaker mode, and go get an AED while you begin CPR.
- Use the AED as soon as it is available.

If someone comes to help and a cell phone is not available

- Ask the person to go phone 9-1-1 and get an AED while you begin CPR.
- Use the AED as soon as it is available.

If you are alone and have a cell phone or nearby phone

- Phone 9-1-1 and put the phone on speaker mode while you begin CPR.
- Give 5 sets of 30 compressions and 2 breaths.
- Go get an AED, and use it as soon as it is available.
- Return to the child and continue CPR.

If you are alone and don't have a cell phone

- Give 5 sets of 30 compressions and 2 breaths.
- Go phone 9-1-1 and get an AED; use the AED as soon as it is available.
- Return to the child and continue CPR.

Provide High-Quality CPR

When providing CPR, give sets of 30 compressions and 2 breaths.

- Make sure the child is lying faceup on a firm, flat surface.
- Quickly move bulky clothes out of the way. If a child's clothes are difficult to remove, you can still provide compressions over clothing.
  - If an AED becomes available, remove all clothes that cover the chest. AED pads must not be placed over any clothing.
- Give 30 chest compressions.
  - Use 1 or 2 hands to give compressions.
    - **1 hand:** Put the heel of one hand on the center of the chest (over the lower half of the breastbone).
    - **2 hands:** Put the heel of one hand on the center of the chest (over the lower half of the breastbone). Put your other hand on top of the first hand.
  - Push straight down at least one third the depth of the chest, or approximately 2 inches.
  - Push at a rate of 100 to 120/min. Count the compressions out loud.
  - Let the chest come back up to its normal position after each compression.
- After 30 compressions, give 2 breaths.
  - Open the airway and give 2 breaths (blow for 1 second for each). Watch for the chest to begin to rise as you give each breath.
  - Try not to interrupt compressions for more than 10 seconds, even when you give breaths.
- Use an AED as soon as it is available.
  - Turn the AED on and follow the prompts.
  - Attach the pads.
    - Use child pads if the child is less than 8 years of age. If child pads are not available, use adult pads.
    - Use adult pads if the child is 8 years or older.
  - Let the AED analyze.
  - Make sure that no one is touching the child, and deliver a shock if advised.
- Provide CPR and use the AED until
  - Someone else arrives who can take turns providing CPR with you
  - The child begins to move, speak, blink, or otherwise react
  - Someone with more advanced training arrives and takes over

Water Safety

Drowning and related injuries are a huge problem, especially for children. However, there are several steps you can personally take to prevent or limit injuries. Any person responsible for children around bodies of water needs to be water competent. *Water competency* is the ability to anticipate, avoid, and survive common drowning situations.

Evidence reveals that many children older than 1 year will benefit from swimming lessons. In contrast, infants, who are younger than 1 year, are developmentally unable to learn the complex movements necessary to swim. But swimming lessons and swimming skills alone cannot prevent all water-related emergencies. Learning to swim needs to be seen as a component of water competency that includes

- Knowing about local hazards and the risks of one's own limitations
- Understanding how to wear a life jacket
- Being able to recognize and respond to a swimmer in distress, shout for help, and perform safe rescue and CPR

Experts generally recommend using multiple layers of protection to prevent drowning because it is unlikely that any single strategy will prevent drowning deaths and injuries. Their recommendations include 5 major evidence-based interventions: 4-sided pool fencing, life jackets, swimming lessons, supervision, and lifeguards.

- **4-sided pool fencing:** Installation of 4-sided fencing (at least 4 feet tall) with self-closing and self-latching gates that completely isolates the pool from the house and yard is the most studied and effective drowning-prevention strategy for young children, preventing more than 50% of swimming-pool drownings of young children.
- **Life jackets:** Life jackets are also well proven to prevent drowning fatalities.
- **Swimming lessons:** Some data reveal that swimming lessons may lower drowning rates among children.
- **Supervision:** Inadequate supervision is often cited as a contributing factor for childhood drowning, especially for younger children. However, adequate supervision, described as close, constant, and attentive supervision of young children in or around any water, is a primary and absolutely essential preventive strategy.
  - For beginning swimmers, adequate supervision is *touch supervision*, in which the supervising adult is within arm's reach of the child so they can pull the child out of the water if the child's head becomes submerged. For more advanced swimmers, supervision should include being capable of recognizing and responding appropriately to a child in distress.
- **Lifeguards:** Lifeguards and CPR training are additional effective preventive measures that can help prevent drowning.

Data about the value of other potential preventive strategies, such as pool covers and pool alarms, are lacking.

Remember, no single factor can eliminate a child's risk of drowning, and a combination of all of these interventions is the best method to minimize drowning. For more information on drowning prevention techniques, visit the American Academy of Pediatrics website at **www.aap.org**.

CPR for Infants

In this section, you will learn when CPR is needed, how to give CPR to an infant, and how to use an AED.

Differences in CPR for Infants vs CPR for Children and Adults

Because infants are so small, there are some differences in how you perform CPR for them compared with what you do for children or adults. When giving chest compressions to an infant, you use only 2 fingers of 1 hand or 2 thumbs—vs 1 or 2 hands for a child and 2 hands for an adult.

Also, for an infant, you should push down about 1½ inches at the rate of 100 to 120/min.

For the purposes of this course, an infant is less than 1 year old.

Assess and Phone 9-1-1

When you see an infant who may have had a cardiac arrest, take the following 5 steps to assess the emergency and get help:

1. Make sure the scene is safe.
2. Tap and shout (check for responsiveness).
3. Shout for help.
4. Check for breathing.
5. Phone 9-1-1, begin CPR, and get an AED.

Depending on the circumstance and resources you have available, you may be able to perform some of these actions at the same time. You might, for example, phone 9-1-1 with your cell phone on speaker mode while checking for breathing.

Step 1: Make Sure the Scene Is Safe

Before you assess the infant, look for anything nearby that might hurt you. You can't help if you get hurt too.

As you help, be aware if anything changes and makes it unsafe for you or the infant.

Step 2: Tap and Shout (Check for Responsiveness)

Actions to Take: Check for Responsiveness
- Tap the infant's foot and shout to check whether they are responsive (Figure 40).
  - If the infant is responsive, continue first aid care.
  - If the infant is unresponsive, shout for help so that if others are nearby, they can help you.

Figure 40. Tap and shout (check for responsiveness).

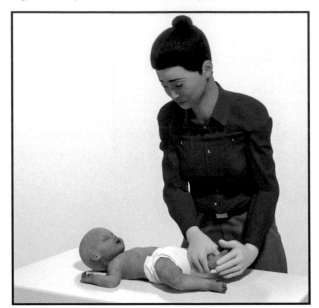

Step 3: Shout for Help

In an emergency, the sooner you realize that there's a problem and get help, the better it is for the infant with a cardiac arrest. When more people are helping, you can provide better care to the infant.

If the infant is unresponsive, shout for help (Figure 41). If someone comes, send that person to phone 9-1-1 and get an AED. If you have a cell phone, phone 9-1-1 and put it on speaker mode.

Figure 41. Shout for help.

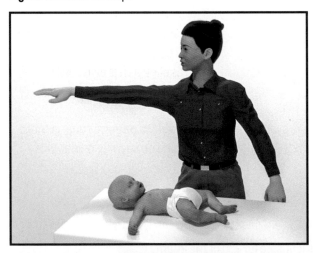

Step 4: Check for Breathing

If the infant is unresponsive, check for breathing (Figure 42). Scan the chest repeatedly for at least 5 seconds (but no more than 10 seconds), looking for the chest to rise and fall. If the infant is not breathing or is only gasping, they need CPR.

Actions to Take: Check for Breathing

If the infant is unresponsive and is breathing

- This infant does not need CPR.
- Roll them onto their side (if you don't suspect a neck or back injury). This will help keep the airway clear in case the infant vomits.
- Stay with the infant until advanced help arrives.

(continued)

Actions to Take: Check for Breathing *(continued)*

If the infant is unresponsive and not breathing or is only gasping

- This infant needs CPR.
- Make sure the infant is lying faceup on a firm, flat surface.
- Have someone phone 9-1-1, or use your cell phone (or nearby phone), put it on speaker mode, and phone 9-1-1.
- Begin CPR. Give 5 sets of 30 compressions and 2 breaths.
- After 5 sets of compressions and breaths, phone 9-1-1 and get an AED (if no one has done this yet). Use the AED as soon as it is available.

Remember: Unresponsive + No breathing or only gasping = Provide CPR

Figure 42. Check for breathing.

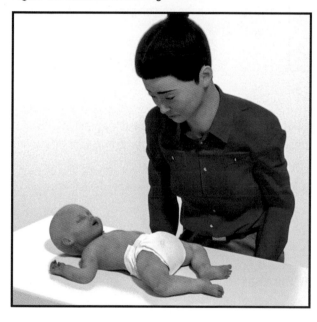

Step 5: Phone 9-1-1, Begin CPR, and Get an AED

If someone comes to help and a cell phone is available

- Ask the person to phone 9-1-1 on the cell phone, put it on speaker mode, and go get an AED while you begin CPR.
- Use the AED as soon as it is available.

If someone comes to help and a cell phone is not available

- Ask the person to go phone 9-1-1 and get an AED while you begin CPR.
- Use the AED as soon as it is available.

If you are alone and have a cell phone or a nearby phone

- Phone 9-1-1 and put the phone on speaker mode while you begin CPR.
- Give 5 sets of 30 compressions and 2 breaths.
- Go get an AED. If the infant isn't injured and you're alone, take the infant with you while you go to phone 9-1-1 and get an AED (Figure 43). Use the AED as soon as it is available.
- Return to the infant and continue CPR.

If you are alone and don't have a cell phone

- Give 5 sets of 30 compressions and 2 breaths.
- Go phone 9-1-1 and get an AED. If the infant isn't injured and you're alone, you can carry the infant with you while you go to phone 9-1-1 and get an AED. Use the AED as soon as it is available.
- Return to the infant and continue CPR.

Figure 43. Take the infant with you while you go to phone 9-1-1 and get an AED.

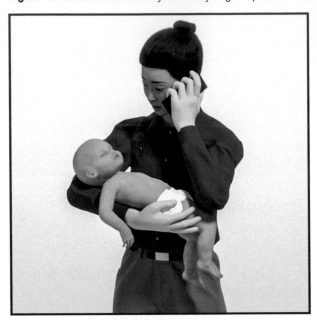

Follow the Dispatcher's Instructions

Stay on the phone until the 9-1-1 dispatcher tells you to hang up. Answering the dispatcher's questions will not delay the arrival of help.

The dispatcher will ask you about the emergency—where you are and what has happened. Dispatchers can provide instructions that will help you, such as telling you how to provide CPR, use an AED, or give first aid.

That's why it's important to put the phone on speaker mode after phoning 9-1-1. It allows the dispatcher and the person providing CPR to speak to each other.

What to Do if You Are Not Sure

It's better to give CPR to an infant who doesn't need it than not to give it to an infant who does need it. CPR is not likely to cause harm if the infant is not in cardiac arrest. But without CPR, an infant who is in cardiac arrest may die.

So if you aren't sure, provide CPR. You may save an infant's life.

Perform High-Quality CPR

Learning how to perform high-quality CPR is important. The better you can perform CPR skills, the better the chances of survival, whether you are helping an adult, a child, or an infant.

CPR Skills

CPR has 2 main skills:

- Providing compressions
- Giving breaths

In this section, you will learn how to perform these skills for an infant in cardiac arrest.

Provide Compressions

You already learned that compressions are the most important part of CPR because they help pump blood to the brain and other organs. Pushing hard and fast when giving compressions is just as important for infants as it is for children and adults.

To perform high-quality CPR, make sure that you

- Provide compressions that are deep enough
- Provide compressions that are fast enough
- Let the chest come back up to its normal position after each compression
- Try not to interrupt compressions for more than 10 seconds, even when you give breaths

Compression depth is an important part of providing high-quality compressions. You need to push hard enough to pump blood through the body. It's better to push too hard than not hard enough. People are often afraid of injuring an infant by providing compressions, but injury is unlikely.

Compression Techniques

Because infants are so much smaller than adults or children, you can use just 2 fingers to provide compressions. Figure 44 shows the correct placement of your fingers on the infant's chest.

Another technique for providing infant chest compressions is to use 2 thumbs. Figure 45 shows the correct placement of your thumbs on the infant's chest.

If you can't provide compressions that are at least one third the depth of the infant's chest, or about 1½ inches, you can use the heel of 1 hand.

Actions to Take: Provide Compressions for an Infant

- Make sure the infant is lying faceup on a firm, flat surface.
- Quickly move bulky clothes out of the way. If an infant's clothes are difficult to remove, you can still provide compressions over clothing.
  - If an AED becomes available, remove all clothes that cover the chest. AED pads must not be placed over any clothing.
- Use 2 fingers, 2 thumbs, or 1 hand to give compressions.
  - **2 fingers:** Place your fingers on the breastbone, just below the nipple line (Figure 44).
  - **2 thumbs:** Place both thumbs side by side on the breastbone, just below the nipple line. Encircle the infant's chest and support the infant's back with the fingers of both hands (Figure 45).
  - **1 hand:** Use the heel of 1 hand to give compressions. Place your hand on the breastbone, just below the nipple line.
- Push straight down at least one third the depth of the chest, or about 1½ inches.
- Push at a rate of 100 to 120/min. Count the compressions out loud.
- Let the chest come back up to its normal position after each compression.

Figure 44. Use 2 fingers of 1 hand to give compressions. Place your fingers on the breastbone, just below the nipple line. Avoid the tip of the breastbone.

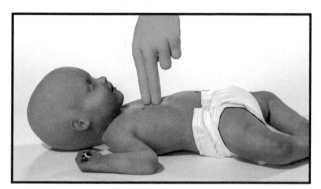

Figure 45. Use 2 thumbs side by side on the breastbone, just below the nipple line. Encircle the infant's chest and support the infant's back with the fingers of both hands.

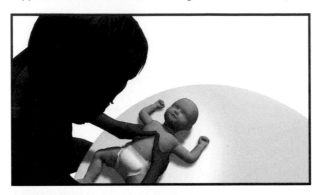

Switch Rescuers to Avoid Fatigue

Performing chest compressions correctly is hard work. The more tired you become, the less effective your compressions will be.

If someone else knows CPR, you can take turns giving compressions. Switch rescuers about every 2 minutes, or sooner if you get tired, moving quickly to keep any pauses in compressions as short as possible.

Remind other rescuers to perform high-quality CPR as described in this section.

Give Breaths

The second skill of CPR is giving breaths. After each set of 30 compressions, you will need to give 2 breaths.

Infants often have healthy hearts, but even an infant's heart can stop beating if they can't breathe or if they have trouble breathing. So it's very important to give breaths as well as compressions to an infant who needs CPR.

Open the Airway

Before giving breaths, open the airway. This lifts the tongue from the back of the throat to make sure your breaths get air into the lungs.

Opening the infant's airway too far can actually close the infant's airway, making it difficult to get air inside. Follow these steps to make sure you open the infant's airway correctly:

> **Actions to Take: Open the Airway**
> - Put one hand on the forehead and the fingers of your other hand on the bony part of the chin. Avoid pressing into the soft part of the neck or under the chin because this might block the airway. Also, don't push the head back too far. This might close the airway as well.
> - Tilt the head back and lift the chin.

Pocket Masks for Giving Breaths

You may give breaths with or without a barrier device, such as a pocket mask. These plastic devices fit over the infant's mouth and nose. They protect the rescuer from blood, vomit, or disease. Your instructor may discuss other types of barrier devices, like face shields, that you can use when giving breaths.

There are different kinds of pocket masks as well as different sizes. So make sure you use the right size for an infant. Pocket masks are typically made of hard plastic with a 1-way valve, which is the part you breathe into. You may need to put a pocket mask together before using it.

Give Breaths Without a Pocket Mask

Giving someone breaths without a barrier device is usually quite safe. Use your best judgment on whether it is safe for you to give breaths.

> **Actions to Take: Give Breaths Without a Pocket Mask**
> - While holding the airway open, take a normal breath. Cover the infant's mouth and nose with your mouth. If you have difficulty making an effective seal, try either a mouth-to-mouth or a mouth-to-nose breath (Figure 46).
>   - If you use the mouth-to-mouth technique, pinch the nose closed.
>   - If you use the mouth-to-nose technique, close the mouth.
> - Give 2 breaths (blow for 1 second for each). Watch for the chest to begin to rise as you give each breath.
> - Try not to interrupt chest compressions for more than 10 seconds, even when you give breaths.

Figure 46. Cover the infant's mouth and nose with your mouth.

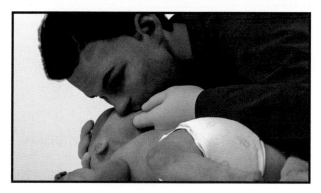

Give Breaths With a Pocket Mask

As you give each breath, look at the infant's chest to see if it begins to rise. For infants, you will not need to blow as much as for larger children. Seeing the chest begin to rise is the best way to know that your breaths are effective.

> **Actions to Take: Give Breaths With a Pocket Mask**
> - Put the mask over the infant's mouth and nose.
>   - If the mask has a narrow, pointed end, put that end of the mask on the bridge of the nose; position the wide end so that it covers the mouth.
> - Tilt the head and lift the chin while pressing the mask against the infant's face. It's important to make an airtight seal between the infant's face and the mask while you lift the chin to keep the airway open (Figure 47).
> - Give 2 breaths (blow for 1 second for each). Watch for the chest to begin to rise as you give each breath.
> - Try not to interrupt chest compressions for more than 10 seconds, even when you give breaths.

Figure 47. Giving breaths with a pocket mask.

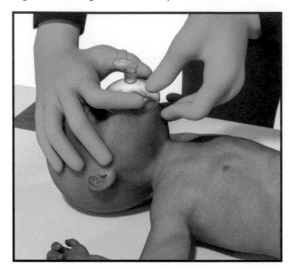

What to Do If the Chest Doesn't Rise

It takes a little practice to give breaths correctly. If you give someone a breath and the chest doesn't rise, do the following:

- Allow the head to go back to its normal position.
- Open the airway again by tilting the head back and lifting the chin.
- Then, give another breath. Make sure the chest rises.

Minimize Interruptions in Chest Compressions

If you have been unable to give 2 effective breaths in 10 seconds, go back to pushing hard and fast on the chest. Try to give breaths again after every 30 compressions.

Don't interrupt compressions for more than 10 seconds.

Actions to Take: Provide Infant CPR

- Make sure the infant is lying faceup on a firm, flat surface.
- Quickly move bulky clothes out of the way. If an infant's clothes are difficult to remove, you can still provide compressions over clothing.
  - If an AED becomes available, remove all clothes that cover the chest. AED pads must not be placed over any clothing.
- Give 30 chest compressions.
  - Use 2 fingers or 2 thumbs of 1 hand to give compressions. Place them on the breastbone, just below the nipple line.
  - Push straight down at least one third the depth of the chest, or about 1½ inches. If you cannot push down this far, you can use the heel of 1 hand to give compressions.
  - Push at a rate of 100 to 120/min. Count the compressions out loud.
  - Let the chest come back up to its normal position after each compression.
- After 30 compressions, give 2 breaths.
  - Open the airway and give 2 breaths (blow for 1 second for each). Watch for the chest to begin to rise as you give each breath.
- Try not to interrupt compressions for more than 10 seconds, even when you give breaths.

Do Not Delay CPR to Get an AED for an Infant

CPR with both compressions and breaths is the most important thing you can do for an infant in cardiac arrest. Do not delay CPR to get an AED for an infant. If someone brings an AED to you, use it as soon as it arrives. See the Use an AED section in CPR and AED Use for Children.

Putting It All Together:
Infant High-Quality CPR Summary

Infants usually have healthy hearts. Often, an infant's heart stops because the infant either can't breathe or is having trouble breathing. For this reason, it's very important to give breaths as well as compressions to an infant.

Compressions are still very important to deliver blood flow, and they are the core of CPR. Try not to interrupt chest compressions for more than 10 seconds when you give breaths.

Assess and Get Help
- Make sure the scene is safe.
- Tap and shout (check for responsiveness).
  - If the infant is responsive, continue first aid care.
  - If the infant is unresponsive, go to the next step.
- Shout for help.
- Check for breathing.
  - If the infant is breathing, stay with the infant until advanced help arrives.
  - If the infant is not breathing or is only gasping, begin CPR and use the AED. See the next steps.

Phone 9-1-1, Begin CPR, and Get an AED

If someone comes to help and a cell phone is available
- Ask the person to phone 9-1-1 on the cell phone, put it on speaker mode, and go get an AED while you begin CPR.
- Use the AED as soon as it is available.

If someone comes to help and a cell phone is not available
- Ask the person to go phone 9-1-1 and get an AED while you begin CPR.
- Use the AED as soon as it is available.

If you are alone and have a cell phone or nearby phone
- Phone 9-1-1 and put the phone on speaker mode while you begin CPR.
- Give 5 sets of 30 compressions and 2 breaths.
- Go get an AED. If the infant isn't injured and you're alone, you can carry the infant with you while you go to phone 9-1-1 and get an AED. Use the AED as soon as it is available.
- Return to the infant and continue CPR.

If you are alone and don't have a cell phone
- Give 5 sets of 30 compressions and 2 breaths.
- Go phone 9-1-1 and get an AED. If the infant isn't injured and you're alone, after 5 sets of 30 compressions and 2 breaths, you can carry the infant with you while you go to phone 9-1-1 and get an AED. Use the AED as soon as it is available.
- Return to the infant and continue CPR.

Provide High-Quality CPR

When providing CPR, give sets of 30 compressions and 2 breaths.

- Make sure the infant is lying faceup on a firm, flat surface.
- Quickly move bulky clothes out of the way. If an infant's clothes are difficult to remove, you can still provide compressions over clothing.
  - If an AED becomes available, remove all clothes that cover the chest. AED pads must not be placed over any clothing.
- Give 30 chest compressions.
  - Use 2 fingers of 1 hand or 2 thumbs to give compressions. Place them on the breastbone, just below the nipple line.
  - Push straight down at least one third the depth of the chest, or about 1½ inches. If you are unable to push down this far, you can use the heel of 1 hand to give compressions.
  - Push at a rate of 100 to 120/min. Count the compressions out loud.
  - Let the chest come back up to its normal position after each compression.
- After 30 compressions, give 2 breaths.
  - Open the airway and give 2 breaths (blow for 1 second for each). Watch for the chest to begin to rise as you give each breath.
  - Try not to interrupt compressions for more than 10 seconds, even when you give breaths.
- Use an AED as soon as it is available.
  - Turn the AED on and follow the prompts.
  - Attach the pads.
    - Use child pads for an infant if available.
    - If child pads are not available, use adult pads.
  - Let the AED analyze.
  - Make sure that no one is touching the infant, and deliver a shock if advised.
- Provide CPR and use the AED until
  - Someone else arrives who can take turns providing CPR with you
  - The infant begins to move, cry, blink, or otherwise react
  - Someone with more advanced training arrives and takes over

Summary of High-Quality CPR Components

Table 3 shows the components of high-quality CPR for each age group.

Table 3. Summary of High-Quality CPR Components

Component	Adult	Children (age 1 year to puberty)	Infants (age less than 1 year)
Make sure the scene is safe	Make sure the scene is safe for you and the person needing help.		
Tap and shout (check for responsiveness)	Check to see if the person is responsive or unresponsive. If unresponsive, go to the next step.		
Shout for help	Shout for help so that if others are nearby, they can help you.		
Check for breathing	If breathing normally, stay with the person until advanced help arrives. If not breathing normally or only gasping, begin CPR and use an AED.	If breathing, stay with the child or infant until advanced help arrives. If not breathing or only gasping, begin CPR and use the AED.	
Phone 9-1-1, begin CPR, and get an AED	Phone or send someone else to phone 9-1-1 and get an AED while you begin CPR. If you are alone and have a phone, put it on speaker mode and phone 9-1-1 while you begin CPR.	Phone or send someone else to phone 9-1-1 and get an AED. If you are alone and have a phone, put it on speaker mode and phone 9-1-1 while you begin CPR. If you are alone and do not have a phone, give 5 sets of 30 compressions and 2 breaths. Then, go phone 9-1-1 and get an AED. Return and continue CPR.	
Compressions and breaths	30 compressions to 2 breaths		
Compression rate	Push on the chest at a rate of 100 to 120/min		
Compression depth	At least 2 inches	At least one third the depth of the chest, or approximately 2 inches	At least one third the depth of the chest, or about 1½ inches
Hand placement	2 hands on the lower half of the breastbone	2 hands or 1 hand (optional for very small child) on the lower half of the breastbone	2 fingers or 2 thumbs in the center of the chest, just below the nipple line; 1 hand if necessary for compression depth
Let the chest come back up	Let the chest come back up to its normal position after each compression		
Minimize interruptions in compressions	Try not to interrupt compressions for more than 10 seconds, even when you give breaths		

Table 4 summarizes the differences in CPR by age group.

Table 4. Differences in CPR for Adults, Infants, and Children

Component	Adult	Children (age 1 year to puberty)	Infants (age less than 1 year)
Compression depth	At least 2 inches	At least one third the depth of the chest, or approximately 2 inches	At least one third the depth of the chest, or about 1½ inches
Hand placement	2 hands on the lower half of the breastbone	2 hands or 1 hand (optional for very small child) on the lower half of the breastbone	2 fingers or 2 thumbs in the center of the chest, just below the nipple line; 1 hand if necessary for compression depth
When to phone 9-1-1 if you are alone and without a phone	After you check breathing, before starting chest compressions	After 5 sets of 30 compressions and 2 breaths	After 5 sets of 30 compressions and 2 breaths; if the infant is uninjured, take the infant with you

Breathing Problems

Sometimes, a person may develop mild or severe blockage of the air passages for many different reasons. One possible cause is asthma, a disease of the air passages. A person who is having an asthma attack will have trouble breathing. Someone experiencing a heart attack, a stroke, or certain injuries also may have breathing problems. Your actions in the first few minutes after you see the signs of any of these conditions could help save a life.

Signs of Breathing Problems

You can tell that someone is having trouble breathing if the person

- Is breathing very fast or very slowly
- Is having trouble with every breath
- Has noisy breathing—you hear a sound or whistle as the air enters or leaves the lungs
- Can only make sounds or speak only a few words at a time between breaths, even though the person is trying to say more

Someone with a medical condition involving breathing problems, such as asthma, usually knows about the condition and what to do. These people often carry inhaler medicine, which helps them breathe more easily within minutes after using it.

At times, a person can have such a hard time breathing that they need help using their inhaler. For this reason, you should be ready to assemble the inhaler and help them use it.

Using an Inhaler

Inhalers have a medicine canister, a mouthpiece, and sometimes a spacer (Figure 48). The spacer can be attached to make it easier for the person with the breathing problem to inhale all the medicine (Figure 49).

Figure 48. Parts of an inhaler: medicine canister, mouthpiece, and spacer.

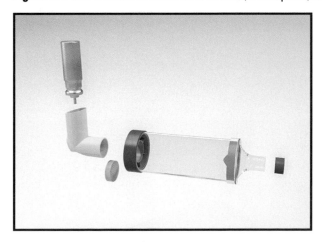

Actions to Take: Use an Inhaler

To use the inhaler

- Remove the cap and shake well.
- Have the person breathe out all the way.
- Place the mouthpiece between their teeth and have them seal their lips around it.
- As they start to breathe in slowly, press down on the canister one time.
- Have them breathe in as slowly and as deeply as they can, for about 5 seconds.
- Count to 10 to allow the medicine to reach the airways of the lung.
- Repeat the steps above for each puff indicated on the inhaler, generally 2 puffs total.
- Replace the cap on the inhaler.

Some inhalers may also come with a separate apparatus called a *spacer* or *chamber*, which is an oval plastic container that attaches to the mouthpiece of the inhaler. If the person's inhaler has a spacer, attach it to the mouthpiece of the inhaler after shaking but before having the person breathe out all the way.

Figure 49. Using an inhaler with a spacer.

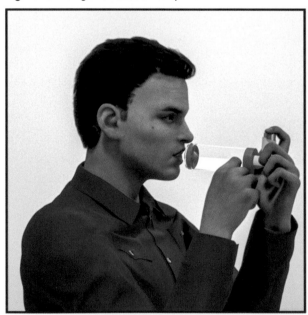

Actions to Take: Help Someone With Breathing Problems

- Ask, "Do you need help?" If the answer is yes, ask "Do you have medicine?"
- If the person has medicine, get it. Then, help the person use it.
- Phone 9-1-1 if the person
  - Has no medicine
  - Does not get better or gets even worse after using their medicine
  - Has trouble speaking
  - Becomes unresponsive
- Stay with the person until someone with more advanced training arrives and takes over.

Choking in an Adult, a Child, or an Infant

Choking is when food or another object gets stuck in the airway in the throat. The object can block the airway and stop air from getting to the lungs. In adults, choking is often caused by food. In children, choking can be caused by food or another object.

Mild vs Severe Airway Block

The block in the airway that causes choking can be either mild or severe. A person with a **mild airway block** can talk or make sounds or can cough loudly. Stand by and let the person cough. If you're worried about the person's breathing, phone 9-1-1.

A person with a **severe airway block** cannot breathe, talk, or make sounds; has a silent cough; or makes the choking sign by holding the neck with 1 or both hands (Figure 50). When this happens, you should act quickly.

Figure 50. The choking sign: holding the neck with 1 or both hands.

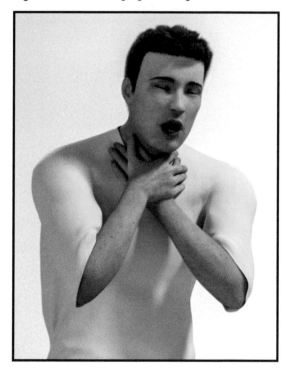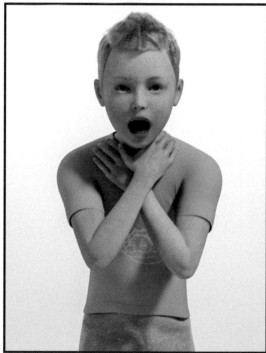

Severe Airway Block in an Adult or a Child

When an adult or a child has a severe airway block, give thrusts slightly above the navel. These thrusts are called *abdominal thrusts*. Each thrust pushes air from the lungs, like a cough does. This can help move or remove an object that is blocking the airway.

Any person who receives abdominal thrusts for choking should see a healthcare provider as soon as possible.

Actions to Take: Severe Airway Block in an Adult or a Child

- If you think someone is choking, ask, "Are you choking? Can I help?"
- If the person nods yes, say, "I'm going to help you."
- Stand firmly or kneel behind the person (depending on your size and the size of the person choking).
- Wrap your arms around the person's waist so that your fists are in front.
- Make a fist with one hand.
- Put the thumb side of your fist slightly above the navel and well below the breastbone.
- Grasp the fist with your other hand and give quick upward thrusts into the abdomen (Figure 51).
- Give thrusts until the object is forced out and the person can breathe, cough, or speak, or until the person becomes unresponsive.

Figure 51. Giving abdominal thrusts.

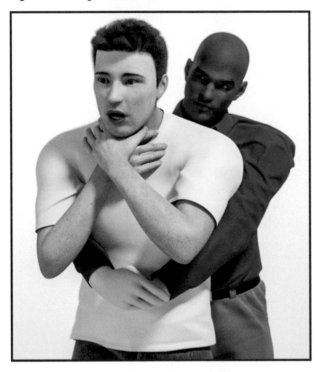 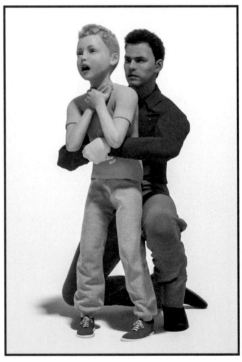

If the person who has a severe airway block is very large or is a pregnant woman, give chest thrusts instead of abdominal thrusts.

Actions to Take: Severe Airway Block in a Pregnant Woman or a Large Adult or Child

- If you can't wrap your arms fully around the waist, give thrusts on the chest instead of the abdomen.
- Put your arms under the armpits and your hands on the lower half of the breastbone.
- Pull straight back to give chest thrusts (Figure 52).

Figure 52. Giving chest thrusts to a choking pregnant woman or a large adult or child.

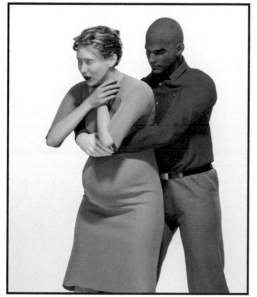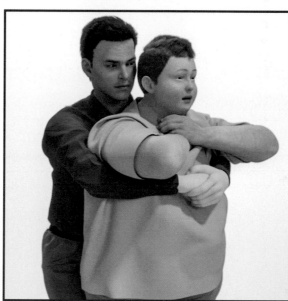

Severe Airway Block in an Infant

When an infant has a severe airway block, use back slaps and chest thrusts to help remove the object. *Give only back slaps and chest thrusts to an infant who is choking.* Never use abdominal thrusts. Giving thrusts to an infant's abdomen can cause serious harm.

Actions to Take: Severe Airway Block in an Infant

- Hold the infant facedown on your forearm. Support the infant's head and jaw with your hand.
- With the heel of your other hand, give up to 5 back slaps between the infant's shoulder blades (Figure 53A).
- If the object does not come out after 5 back slaps, turn the infant over, supporting the head.
- Give up to 5 chest thrusts, using 2 fingers of your other hand to push on the chest in the same place you push during CPR (Figure 53B).
- Repeat giving 5 back slaps and 5 chest thrusts until the infant can breathe, cough, or cry, or until they become unresponsive.

Figure 53. How to help an infant who has a severe airway block. **A,** Back slaps. **B,** Chest thrusts.

A

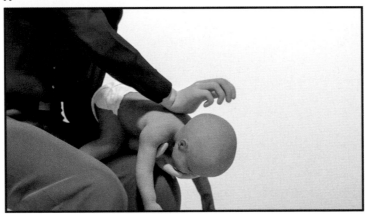

B

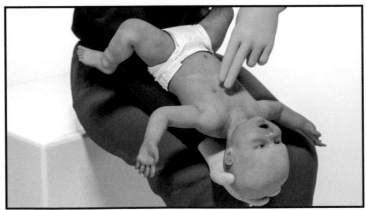

Help a Choking Adult, Child, or Infant Who Becomes Unresponsive

If you can't remove the object blocking the airway, the person will become unresponsive. Always give CPR to anyone who is unresponsive and is not breathing normally or is only gasping. Giving both compressions and breaths is very important for someone with a severe airway block who becomes unresponsive.

Review how to provide CPR and use an AED in the CPR and AED section.

Remember: Unresponsive + No breathing or only gasping = Provide CPR

Choking Adult Who Becomes Unresponsive

Actions to Take: Help a Choking Adult Who Becomes Unresponsive

- Shout for help.
- Phone or have someone else phone 9-1-1 and get an AED. Put the phone on speaker mode so that you can talk to the dispatcher.
- Provide CPR, starting with compressions.
- After each set of 30 compressions, open the airway to give breaths.
- Look in the mouth. If you see an object in the mouth, take it out.
- Give 2 breaths and then repeat 30 compressions.
- Continue CPR until
  - The person moves, speaks, blinks, or otherwise reacts
  - Someone with more advanced training arrives and takes over

Remember: Every time you open the airway to give breaths, look for the object in the back of the throat. If you see an object, take it out.

Do not perform a blind finger sweep. This could cause the object to get lodged farther back in the airway.

Choking Child or Infant Who Becomes Unresponsive

A child or an infant who has a severe airway block and becomes unresponsive needs immediate CPR. If you are alone without a cell phone, it is important to provide 5 sets of 30 compressions and 2 breaths first. Then, you can leave the child or infant, or carry the child or infant with you, while you go to phone 9-1-1 and get an AED. Use the AED as soon as it is available.

Actions to Take: Help a Choking Child or Infant Who Becomes Unresponsive

- Shout for help.
- Make sure the child or infant is lying faceup on a firm, flat surface.
- Phone 9-1-1, begin CPR, and get an AED. Use the AED as soon as it is available.

If someone comes to help and a cell phone is available

- Ask the person to phone 9-1-1 on the cell phone, put it on speaker mode, and go get an AED while you begin CPR.
- Use the AED as soon as it is available.

If someone comes to help and a cell phone is not available

- Ask the person to phone 9-1-1 and go get an AED while you begin CPR.
- Use the AED as soon as it is available.

(continued)

Actions to Take: Help a Choking Child or Infant Who Becomes Unresponsive *(continued)*

If you are alone and do have a cell phone

- Phone 9-1-1 and put the phone on speaker mode while you begin CPR.
- Give 5 sets of 30 compressions and 2 breaths.
- Go get an AED, and use it as soon as it is available. (If you're alone, you can carry the child or infant with you while you go to get an AED.)
- Return to the child or infant and continue CPR.

If you are alone and don't have a cell phone

- Give 5 sets of 30 compressions and 2 breaths.
- Phone 9-1-1 and get an AED. Use the AED as soon as it is available. (If you're alone, you can carry the child or infant with you while you go to phone 9-1-1 and get an AED.)
- Return to the child or infant and continue CPR.
- Provide CPR.
    - Give sets of 30 compressions and 2 breaths.
    - After each set of 30 compressions, open the airway to give breaths.
    - Look in the mouth (Figure 54). If you see an object in the mouth, take it out. *Do not perform a blind finger sweep.*
    - Give 2 breaths.
- Continue CPR and looking in the mouth after each set of compressions until
    - The child or infant moves, cries, speaks, blinks, or otherwise reacts.
    - Someone with more advanced training arrives and takes over.

Figure 54. Look in the mouth for objects.

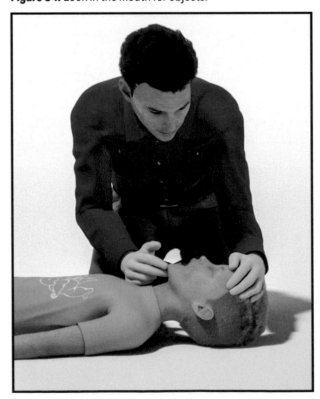

Allergic Reactions

Allergies are quite common, but for some people, certain things can cause a severe allergic reaction that can quickly turn into a medical emergency. Signs of a mild allergic reaction include stuffy nose, sneezing, itching around the eyes or on the skin, and a raised, red rash on the skin (hives).

Signs of a severe allergic reaction include trouble breathing, swelling of the tongue or face, or signs of shock.

Some things that can cause a severe allergic reaction are

- Chocolate
- Eggs
- Insect bites and stings, especially bee stings
- Peanuts
- Some medications

Epinephrine Pen for a Severe Allergic Reaction

Epinephrine is a drug that can stop a severe allergic reaction. It is available by prescription in a self-injectable device called an *epinephrine pen.* People who are known to have severe allergic reactions are encouraged to carry epinephrine pens with them at all times.

There are 2 types of epinephrine pens: spring activated and electronic. They are different for children and adults, so be sure you are using the person's prescribed device.

Usually, a person who has an epinephrine pen will know how and when to use it. If the person needs help administering an epinephrine injection and they have a prescription, Good Samaritan laws allow for you to help, providing you act in good faith.

Actions to Take: Use an Epinephrine Pen

- Follow the instructions on the pen. The needle comes out of one end of the pen, so always hold the pen in your fist without touching either end. You can give the injection through clothes or on bare skin.
- Take off the safety cap (Figure 55A).
- Hold the leg firmly in place just before and during the injection. Press the tip of the injector hard against the side of the person's thigh, about halfway between the hip and the knee (Figure 55B).
  - Different injectors need to be held in place for different amounts of time. Be familiar with the manufacturer's instructions for the type of injector you are using. For example, EpiPen and EpiPen Jr injectors recommend holding the injector in place for 3 seconds. Some other injectors recommend holding them in place for up to 10 seconds.
- Pull the pen straight out, making sure you don't touch the end that was pressed against the person's thigh.
- Either the person getting the injection or the person giving the injection should rub the injection spot for about 10 seconds.
- Note the time of the injection.
- If the person doesn't get better, phone 9-1-1. If it takes more than 10 minutes for advanced help to arrive, consider giving a second dose, if available.
- Give any used pens to the emergency responders for proper disposal.

Figure 55. Using an epinephrine pen. **A,** Take off the safety cap. **B,** Press the tip of the injector hard against the side of the person's thigh, about halfway between the hip and the knee.

A

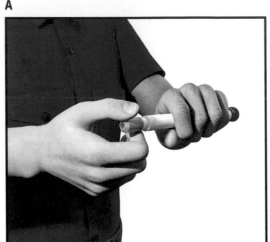

B

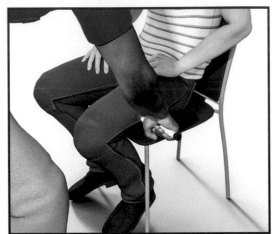

Dispose of the Epinephrine Pen Correctly

It's important to dispose of needles correctly so that no one gets stuck. Follow your company's disposal policy for sharps. If you don't know what to do, give the needle to someone with more advanced training.

If possible, save a sample of what caused the reaction.

Heart Attack

Heart disease is one of the leading causes of death in the world.

If someone has signs of a possible heart attack, you must act and phone 9-1-1 right away—even if the person doesn't want you to. The first minutes of a heart attack are the most important. That's when a person is likely to get worse or even die. Also, many treatments for heart attack are most successful if you give them quickly.

If a person says they have chest pain, make sure they stay calm and rest. It's best if the person doesn't drive themselves to the hospital. Stay with them until someone with more advanced training arrives and takes over.

Difference Between Heart Attack and Cardiac Arrest

People often use the terms *cardiac arrest* and *heart attack* to mean the same thing—but they are not the same. *Cardiac arrest* is a "rhythm" problem. It occurs when the heart malfunctions and stops beating unexpectedly. A *heart attack* is a "clot" problem. It occurs when a clot blocks blood flow.

Cardiac Arrest

Cardiac arrest results from an abnormal heart rhythm. This abnormal rhythm causes the heart to quiver so that it can no longer pump blood to the brain, lungs, and other organs. Within seconds, the person becomes unresponsive and is not breathing or is only gasping. Death occurs within minutes if the victim does not receive immediate lifesaving treatment.

Heart Attack

A heart attack occurs when blood flow to part of the heart muscle is blocked by a clot. Typically during a heart attack, the heart continues to pump blood. The longer the person with a heart attack goes without treatment, the greater the possible damage to the heart muscle. Occasionally, the damaged heart muscle triggers an abnormal rhythm that can lead to cardiac arrest.

Signs of a Heart Attack

- **Chest discomfort:** Most heart attacks involve discomfort in the center of the chest that lasts more than a few minutes or that goes away and comes back. It can feel like uncomfortable pressure, squeezing, fullness, or pain. It may be mistaken for heartburn or indigestion.
- **Discomfort in other areas of the body:** Discomfort also may appear in other areas of the upper body. Symptoms can include pain or discomfort in one or both arms or in the back, neck, jaw, shoulder, or stomach.
- **Other signs:** Other signs of a heart attack are shortness of breath (with or without chest discomfort), breaking out in a cold sweat, nausea, or light-headedness.

Signs in Women

Women may be more likely than men to experience these signs of a heart attack:

- An uncomfortable feeling in the back, jaw, neck, or shoulder
- Shortness of breath
- Nausea or vomiting

Admitting Discomfort

Many people won't admit that their discomfort may be caused by a heart attack. People often say the following:

- "I'm too healthy."
- "I don't want to bother the doctor."
- "I don't want to frighten my spouse."
- "I'll feel silly if it isn't a heart attack."

If you suspect someone is having a heart attack, act quickly and phone 9-1-1 right away. Don't hesitate, even if the person doesn't want to admit discomfort.

Actions to Take: Signs of a Heart Attack

- Make sure the person stays calm and rests. Phone or have someone else phone 9-1-1.
- Ask someone to get the first aid kit and an AED if available.
- If the person doesn't have an allergy to aspirin, serious bleeding, or signs of a stroke, have them chew and swallow 1 full-strength (adult) aspirin or 2 low-dose aspirins.
  - If you are uncertain about the person's allergies or uncomfortable giving aspirin, do not encourage the person to take aspirin.
- If the person becomes unresponsive, be prepared to give CPR and use the AED.

Heart Attack Symptoms:
Men vs Women

The most common symptom of a heart attack for both men and women is chest pain. But women may experience less obvious warning signs.

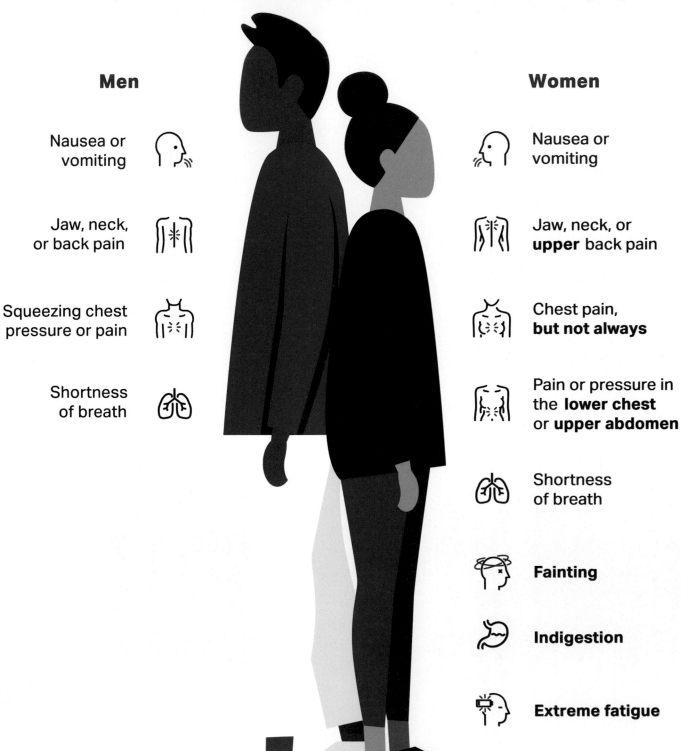

Men

Nausea or vomiting

Jaw, neck, or back pain

Squeezing chest pressure or pain

Shortness of breath

Women

Nausea or vomiting

Jaw, neck, or **upper** back pain

Chest pain, **but not always**

Pain or pressure in the **lower chest** or **upper abdomen**

Shortness of breath

Fainting

Indigestion

Extreme fatigue

Source: American Heart Association's journal, *Circulation*

Fainting

Fainting is a short period of time, usually less than a minute, when a person briefly stops responding and then seems fine. Often, a person who faints gets dizzy and then becomes unresponsive. Fainting may occur when someone

- Stands without moving for a long time, especially if it's hot
- Has a heart condition
- Suddenly stands after squatting or bending down
- Receives bad news

There are also certain movements someone can do that will help prevent fainting (Figure 56).

Figure 56. How to help prevent fainting. **A,** Help the person lie flat on the floor. **B,** Don't let them get up too quickly. **C,** Have them put their head between their legs if they are sitting.

A

B

C

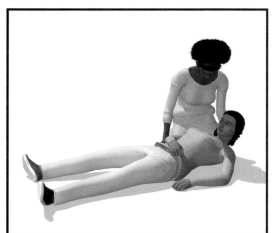 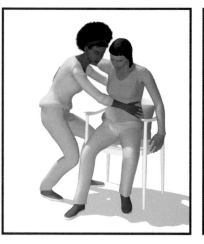 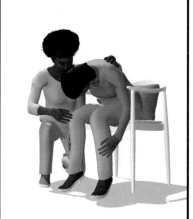

Actions to Take: Prevent Someone From Fainting or Help Someone Who Is Dizzy but Still Responds

- Help the person lie flat on the floor.
- Don't let them get up too quickly.
- Put their head between their knees if they are sitting.
- If the person is lying down, have them cross one leg over the other and tense their leg, abdominal, and buttocks muscles.
- You can also have them lower their body into a squatting position and tense their abdominal muscles.
- Phone 9-1-1 if the person doesn't improve or becomes unresponsive.
- If the person becomes unresponsive and is not breathing, give CPR.

Actions to Take: Help Someone Who Faints

- Make sure the person is on their back.
- Make sure the person is breathing and has no injuries.
- If the person stays unresponsive for more than 1 minute, phone 9-1-1.
- Do not move the injured person if you suspect a head, neck, or spine injury.

If the person starts to respond

- Ask the person to continue to lie flat on the floor until they can sit up and feel normal.
- If the person fell, look for injuries caused by the fall.
- Phone 9-1-1.

Diabetes and Low Blood Sugar

Diabetes is a disease that affects the levels of sugar in the blood. Too much or too little sugar causes problems. Some people with diabetes take medication, such as insulin, to maintain their sugar levels. Low blood sugar can occur if someone with diabetes has not eaten or is vomiting, has not eaten enough food for the level of activity, or has injected too much insulin.

Signs of Low Blood Sugar in a Person With Diabetes

If the person's blood sugar does get too low, behavior can change. Signs of low blood sugar can come on quickly. When a person with diabetes has low blood sugar, the person may become

- Irritable or confused
- Hungry or weak
- Sleepy
- Sweaty

In some cases, the person might even have a seizure.

Actions to Take: Signs of Low Blood Sugar

If the person can't sit up or swallow

- Phone or have someone else phone 9-1-1. Do not try to give the person anything to eat or drink.

If the person can sit up and swallow

- Ask the person to eat or drink something with sugar that can rapidly restore blood glucose levels. These items include glucose tablets, orange juice, soft chewy candy, jelly beans, or fruit leather.
- Have the person sit quietly or lie down.
- If the person does not improve within 10 minutes, phone or have someone else phone 9-1-1.

Stroke

Stroke is another medical emergency for which you may need to use your first aid skills. Strokes occur when blood stops flowing to a part of the brain. This can happen if a blood vessel in the brain is blocked or leaks.

For many people, getting treatment in the first hours after a stroke can reduce the damage and improve recovery. So it's important to recognize the signs of stroke quickly and get immediate medical care.

Warning Signs of Stroke

Use the F.A.S.T. method to recognize and remember the warning signs of stroke (Figure 57). *F.A.S.T.* stands for face, arms, speech, and time.

F Face drooping: Does one side of the face droop, or is it numb?

A Arm weakness: Is one arm weak or numb?

S Speech difficulty: Is speech slurred?

T Time to phone 9-1-1: If someone shows any of these symptoms, phone 9-1-1 immediately.

Figure 57. Use the F.A.S.T. method to remember the warning signs of stroke.

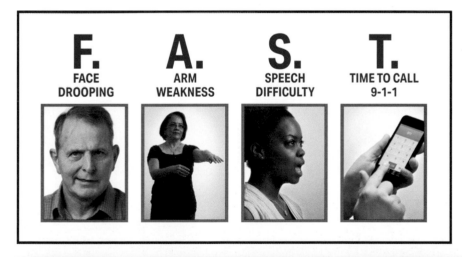

Actions to Take: Stroke
- Phone or have someone else phone 9-1-1 and get the first aid kit and AED.
- Note the time when the stroke signs first appeared.
- Remain with the person until someone with more advanced training arrives and takes over.
- If the person becomes unresponsive and is not breathing normally or is only gasping, give CPR.

Seizure

A *seizure* is abnormal electrical activity in the brain. Seizures are often caused by a medical condition called *epilepsy,* and they usually stop within a few minutes. Seizures also can be caused by head injury, low blood sugar, heat-related injury, poisoning, or cardiac arrest.

Signs of a Seizure

Signs of a seizure may differ. Some people who are having a seizure may

- Lose muscle control
- Fall to the ground
- Stop responding
- Have jerking movements of the arms, legs, and sometimes other parts of the body

However, not all seizures look like this. Other people might become unresponsive and have a glassy-eyed stare.

During the seizure, a person may bite their tongue, cheek, or mouth. You can give first aid for that injury when the seizure is over. After a seizure, the person might be confused, slow to respond, or even fall asleep.

Caution

If someone is having a seizure, don't put anything in the person's mouth. This can actually hurt instead of help. The most important first aid action you can take for a person having a seizure is to protect them from injury.

Actions to Take: During a Seizure
- Move furniture or other objects out of the way.
- Place something soft under the person's head.
- Never hold the person down or put something in their mouth.

Actions to Take: After a Seizure
- Quickly check to see if the person is responsive and breathing.
- Stay with the person until someone with more advanced training arrives and takes over.
- If the person is having trouble breathing because of vomiting or fluids in their mouth, roll them onto their side.
- If they are unresponsive and are not breathing normally or are only gasping, give CPR.

Bleeding From the Mouth

If the person has bitten their tongue, cheek, or mouth and is bleeding, give first aid after the seizure. See the Bleeding From the Mouth section in Injury Emergencies.

Medical Emergencies: Review Questions

1. When giving abdominal thrusts to an adult who is choking, you should
    a. Place your hands near the throat
    b. Place your hands near the left side of the lower abdomen
    c. Put the thumb side of your fist slightly above their navel and well below the breastbone

2. Signs of a severe allergic reaction include trouble breathing or swelling of the face and tongue, and the person may stop responding.
    a. True
    b. False

3. A person with a _____ is usually awake and can talk but may have an uncomfortable feeling, such as pain or pressure, in the chest.
    a. Stroke
    b. Seizure
    c. Heart attack

4. The warning signs of _____ include sudden numbness or weakness of the face, arm, or leg, especially on one side of the body.
    a. Fainting
    b. Stroke
    c. Heart attack
    d. Seizure

5. If someone with low blood sugar is responding and can sit up and swallow, give the person something that contains sugar to eat or drink.
    a. True
    b. False

6. For high-quality adult CPR, you should push
    a. At a rate of 80 to 100 compressions per minute
    b. At a rate of no more than 60 compressions per minute
    c. At a rate of 100 to 120 compressions per minute

7. What is the first link in the adult Chain of Survival?
    a. Early CPR
    b. Rapid AED use
    c. Recognizing the emergency

8. When you phone 9-1-1, you should
   a. Answer all the dispatcher's questions
   b. Tell the dispatcher to call you back
   c. Give the dispatcher only the victim's information

9. If someone isn't breathing or responding, you should start CPR and use an AED if available.
   a. True
   b. False

10. What is a sign that an infant is not responding?
    a. The infant cries and blinks
    b. The infant does nothing when you tap and shout

11. How deep should you push for adult chest compressions?
    a. One half the depth of the chest
    b. One third the depth of the chest
    c. At least 2 inches

12. When performing CPR, you should switch positions
    a. About every 2 minutes
    b. About every 5 minutes
    c. About every 10 minutes

13. To give breaths with a mask, tilt the head and cover the face completely with the mask.
    a. True
    b. False

14. If you are providing CPR and another person arrives with an AED, you should use it immediately.
    a. True
    b. False

15. How deep should you push for child chest compressions?
    a. Approximately 2 inches
    b. About 1 inch
    c. About half an inch

16. If you are performing CPR on a child and the AED has only adult pads, what should you do?
    a. Don't use the AED because the pads are only for adults
    b. Use the adult pads, making sure they do not touch each other
    c. Place the AED pads over the clothing to reduce the shock

17. If you are alone with an uninjured infant who needs CPR, give 5 sets of 30 compressions and 2 breaths, and then
    a. Check for breathing
    b. See if someone can help
    c. Carry the infant with you while you go to phone 9-1-1

18. How deep should you push for infant chest compressions?
    a. As far as possible without breaking any of the infant's ribs
    b. At least one third the depth of the chest, or about 1½ inches

19. If a child is choking, you should put 2 fingers above their navel to give abdominal thrusts.
    a. True
    b. False

20. If an infant is still choking after you've given 5 back slaps and 5 chest thrusts, you should
    a. Repeat back slaps and chest thrusts until the infant can breathe or stops responding
    b. Put a finger in the infant's mouth and attempt to remove the blockage

Answers:

1. c, 2. a, 3. c, 4. b, 5. a, 6. c, 7. c, 8. a, 9. a, 10. b, 11. c, 12. a, 13. b, 14. a, 15. a, 16. b, 17. c, 18. b, 19. b, 20. a

Injury Emergencies

For any injury emergency, your first steps will be to make sure the scene is safe, get the first aid kit, and put on PPE.

External Bleeding

Minor bleeding occurs from small cuts or scrapes. With all bleeding injuries, your first action should be to identify 2 factors to guide your care:

- The amount of bleeding
- The location of the bleeding

Minor bleeding is easily controlled, often with a simple adhesive bandage. For minor cuts anywhere on the body, wash the area with soap and water, and then apply a dressing to the wound. Once the bleeding has stopped, you can apply an antibiotic ointment, if the person has no known allergies, and an adhesive bandage. This method has been proven to help wounds heal faster and more effectively.

If the wound is bleeding more than can easily be stopped with an adhesive bandage, you will need to determine whether it is non–life-threatening or life-threatening bleeding.

Consider a wound to be life-threatening if the flow of blood is continuous and steady and if the volume of loss appears large, about equal to half of a 12-ounce can. You do not want to wait for blood to accumulate to take action because cuts that may seem more moderate at first can become severe if the person is on certain types of blood-thinning medications, like aspirin. It is important to not underestimate the amount of blood loss; be prepared to take action.

Phone or ask someone else to phone 9-1-1 if

- There is a lot of bleeding
- You cannot stop the bleeding
- You see signs of shock
- You suspect a head, neck, or spine injury
- You are not sure what to do

Direct Pressure and Bandaging

Many people confuse the terms *dressing* and *bandage*. Here is what they mean and how they work together:

- A *dressing* is a clean material used directly on a wound to stop bleeding. It can be a piece of gauze or any other clean piece of cloth.
- A *bandage* is material used to protect or cover an injured body part. A bandage can also be used to help keep pressure on a wound.

If necessary, you can hold gauze dressings in place over a wound with a bandage (Figure 58).

Figure 58. Using dressings and a bandage on a wound. **A,** Apply dressings over the bleeding area, and put direct pressure on the dressings. Use the heel of your hand to apply pressure directly to the wound. **B,** Place a bandage over the dressings.

A

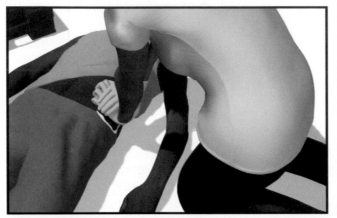

B

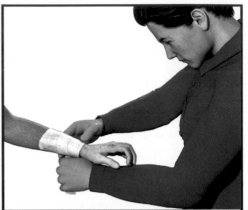

Actions to Take: Control Non–Life-Threatening Bleeding With Direct Pressure and Bandaging

- Apply dressings over the bleeding area, and put direct pressure on the dressings.
  - Use the heel of your hand to apply pressure directly to the wound.
- If the bleeding is not life-threatening, apply a dressing to the bleeding area.
  - Put direct pressure on the dressings by using the heel of one hand, with the other hand stacked on top of the first. If possible, keep your arms straight while applying pressure downward onto the wound. Direct pressure should be firm, steady, and constant.
- Do not remove pressure from the wound to add more dressings. Also, do not remove a dressing once it's in place because this could cause the wound to bleed more. Continue holding firm pressure until help arrives or the bleeding stops. Releasing pressure too soon can allow the wound to start bleeding again.
- If the bleeding does not stop, press harder. Keep pressure on the wound until it stops bleeding.
- Once the bleeding stops, or if you cannot keep pressure on the wound, wrap a bandage firmly over the dressings to hold them in place.
- A person who is bleeding should be seen by a healthcare provider as soon as possible because the person may need stitches or a tetanus shot.

Tourniquet

If the person has severe bleeding on an arm or a leg, you'll need to use a tourniquet. Because uncontrolled bleeding can lead to more complications, phone 9-1-1 and get an AED, if one is available. Life-threatening bleeding can occur from a variety of traumatic injuries, such as car accidents, cuts from glass, accidents involving saws or other tools, knife penetration injuries, gunshot wounds, or falls from a height. You should always phone 9-1-1 first when there is life-threatening bleeding.

The first aid kit should contain a premade or manufactured tourniquet. If it doesn't, we recommend adding it to your kit, especially if your workplace meets the requirements of Class B locations. If applied correctly, a tourniquet should stop the bleeding. Tightening the tourniquet may cause pain, but it will minimize blood loss.

Actions to Take: Use a Manufactured Tourniquet

- Apply the tourniquet 2 to 3 inches above the bleeding site.
- Do not place the tourniquet on a joint.
- Pull the free end of the tourniquet to make it as tight as possible, and then secure it.
- Twist the windlass, or knob, until the bleeding stops.
- You need to twist the windlass as tight as possible to stop the life-threatening bleeding. This may cause the person discomfort or pain.
- Secure the windlass in the clip and note the time the tourniquet was applied.

For more information on how to use a premade tourniquet, see Figure 59.

Figure 59. Using a manufactured tourniquet. **A,** Put direct pressure on the dressings using the heel of one hand, with the other hand stacked on top of the first. Direct pressure should be firm, steady, and constant. **B,** Apply the tourniquet 2 to 3 inches above the bleeding site on the person's arm or leg, closer to the heart. **C,** Pull the free end of the tourniquet to make it as tight as possible, and then secure it. **D,** Twist the windlass, or knob, as tight as possible until the bleeding stops. **E,** Secure the windlass and note the time the tourniquet was applied.

A

B

C

D

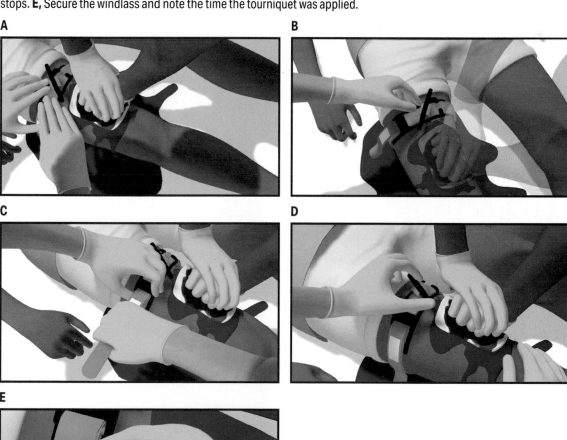

E

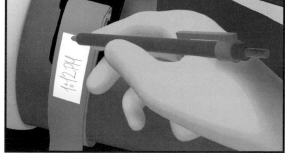

If you do not have a manufactured tourniquet or if one fails to stop bleeding, apply direct pressure with a hemostatic dressing, if available. A *hemostatic dressing* is a wound dressing that contains an agent that promotes blood clotting. If direct pressure with or without a hemostatic dressing fails to stop the life-threatening bleeding, a first aid provider trained in the use of an improvised tourniquet may consider using one.

If the bleeding is severe and is located on a body part that is not the arm or leg, such as the head, neck, chest, abdomen, shoulders, or hips, you can pack the wound and then apply pressure as noted above. *Packing the wound* means to take a material like gauze or clothing and place it tightly into the wound (Figure 60). You would then apply pressure and a compression dressing.

Figure 60. Packing the wound. **A,** Pack the wound with gauze or a clean cloth. **B,** Place it tightly in the wound. **C,** Continue to apply direct pressure until the bleeding stops.

A

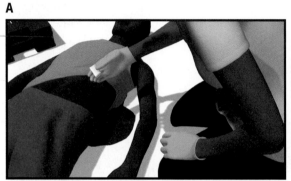

B

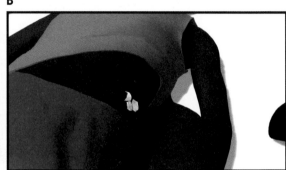

C

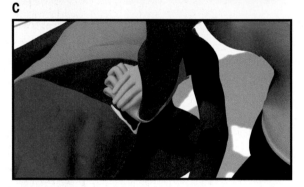

Shock

Losing a large amount of blood can lead to a life-threatening condition called *shock.* Shock happens when the body's tissues and organs are not getting enough blood. Besides loss of blood from a severe injury, shock can be caused by other types of emergencies, such as a heart attack or a severe allergic reaction. An injury that causes internal bleeding can also lead to shock.

Signs of Shock

A person in shock may

- Feel weak, faint, or dizzy
- Feel nauseated or thirsty
- Have pale or grayish skin
- Be restless, agitated, or confused
- Be cold and clammy to the touch

Actions to Take: Shock

- Phone 9-1-1 and get the first aid kit and AED, if available.
- Help the person lie down on their back.
- Cover the person with a blanket to keep them warm.
- Check to see if CPR is needed. If so, give CPR.

Wounds

Wounds are common first aid emergencies. A *wound* is an injury of the soft tissue in the body. Wounds can range from minor injuries, such as scrapes and small cuts, to more serious ones, such as penetrating wounds.

Bleeding From the Nose

A person with a nosebleed should lean forward, not backward. Leaning backward will not help stop the bleeding. You will see less blood when a person leans back because the blood drains down the throat. But swallowed blood can lead to vomiting.

Actions to Take: Nosebleed

- Have the person sit down and lean forward.
- Pinch the soft part of the nose on both sides (Figure 61) with a clean dressing.
- Place constant pressure on the nostrils for a few minutes until the bleeding stops. If bleeding continues, press harder.
- Phone 9-1-1 if
  - You can't stop the bleeding in about 15 minutes
  - The bleeding is heavy, such as gushing blood
  - The injured person has trouble breathing

Figure 61. Press on both sides of the nostrils.

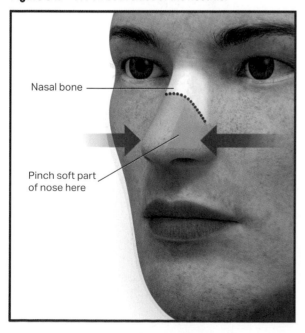

Nasal bone

Pinch soft part of nose here

Bleeding From the Mouth

Bleeding from the mouth can usually be stopped with pressure. If a mouth injury is severe, blood or broken teeth can block the airway and cause breathing problems.

Actions to Take: Control Bleeding From the Mouth

- If bleeding is coming from the tongue, lip, or cheek and you can reach it easily, apply pressure with gauze or a clean cloth (Figure 62).
- If you haven't phoned 9-1-1 and you can't stop the bleeding in 5 to 10 minutes, or if the person has trouble breathing, phone or ask someone else to phone 9-1-1.

Figure 62. If the bleeding is from the tongue, lip, or cheek, press the bleeding area with sterile gauze or a clean cloth.

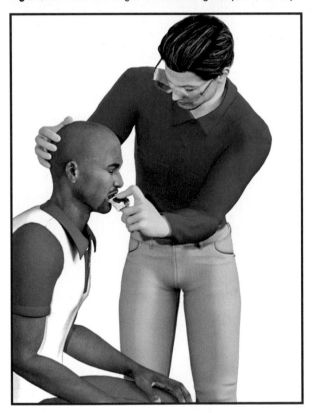

Tooth Injuries

Sometimes when a person suffers a mouth injury, one or more teeth may be broken, loosened, or knocked out. This can be a choking hazard.

Actions to Take: Tooth Injury

- Check the person's mouth for any missing or loose teeth or parts of teeth.
  - If a tooth is chipped, gently clean the injured area and contact a dentist.
  - If a tooth is loose, have the person bite down on a piece of gauze to keep the tooth in place, and contact a dentist.
  - If a tooth has come out, a dentist may be able to reattach the tooth. So when you hold it, hold it by the crown—the top part of the tooth (Figure 63). Do not hold it by the root.
- Apply pressure with gauze to stop any bleeding in the empty tooth socket.
- Clean the area where the tooth was located with saline or clean water.
- Put the tooth in an oral rehydration salt solution, or wrap the tooth in cling film.
  - As a last resort, you can store the tooth in cow's milk or the injured person's saliva—but not in the mouth. Do not store the tooth in tap water.
- Immediately take the injured person and the tooth to a dentist or emergency department.

Figure 63. Hold the tooth by the crown.

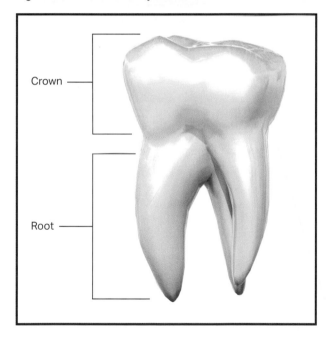

Crown

Root

Eye Injuries

A direct hit to the eye or a chemical in the eye can create big problems. If the eye is hit hard or punctured, phone 9-1-1 and tell the person to keep both eyes closed.

Signs of an eye injury include

- Pain
- Trouble seeing
- Bruising
- Bleeding
- Redness or swelling

Actions to Take: Eye Injury

- If something small like sand gets in a person's eye, rinse with lots of running water.
- Tell the person not to rub their eye.
- Phone 9-1-1 if
  - The sand or object doesn't come out
  - The person has extreme pain
  - The person still has trouble seeing
- Tell the person to keep their eyes closed until someone with more advanced training arrives and takes over.

Actions to Take: Chemical Eye Injury

- Rinse the eyes with lots of water (Figure 64). Rinse for at least 15 minutes or until someone with more advanced training arrives and takes over.
  - If an eyewash station or kit is nearby, use it.
  - If neither is available, use water from the tap or normal saline or contact lens solution.
    - *Caution:* If only one eye is affected, make sure the eye with the chemicals in it is the lower eye as you rinse. Try not to rinse the chemicals into the unaffected eye.
- Contact your local poison control center or, if a poison control center is not available, seek help from a medical provider or phone 9-1-1.

Figure 64. Help the person wash their eyes and face under water flowing from a faucet or hose, or use an eyewash station.

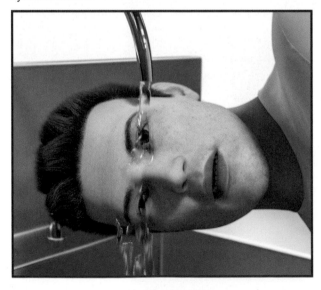

Penetrating and Puncturing Injuries

An object such as a knife, nail, or sharp stick can wound a person by puncturing the skin or penetrating the body. If the object is stuck in the body, leave it there until a healthcare provider can treat the injury. Taking it out may cause more bleeding and damage.

Actions to Take: Penetrating or Puncturing Injury

- Phone 9-1-1 and get the first aid kit and AED.
- Try to keep the injured person from moving.
- Put on gloves, and try to stop any bleeding you can see.
- If the object is stuck in the body, leave it there.
- Be prepared to give CPR and use the AED if the person becomes unresponsive and stops breathing.

Amputation

Amputation occurs when any part of an arm or leg is cut or torn off.

A traumatic amputation may seem overwhelming, but you need to act quickly. Your first action should be to stop the bleeding by using a tourniquet or direct pressure. Then, you can take steps to protect the amputated part, which is also important because surgeons may be able to reattach amputated fingers or toes.

Actions to Take: Control Bleeding From Amputation

- Make sure the scene is safe.
- Phone 9-1-1 and get the first aid kit and AED.
- Use a tourniquet to stop the bleeding (refer to the External Bleeding section for details on how to use a tourniquet).
- If a tourniquet is unavailable, or if does not stop the bleeding, apply dressings from the first aid kit and put direct pressure on the dressings over the bleeding area.

Actions to Take: Protect an Amputated Part

- Rinse the amputated part with clean water (Figure 65A).
- Cover it with a clean dressing.
- Place it in a watertight plastic bag (Figure 65B).
- Place that bag inside a separate container that contains ice or ice water (Figure 65C). Label it with the injured person's name, the date, and the time.
- Make sure the body part gets to the hospital with the injured person. *Remember:* Do not place the amputated body part directly on ice.

Figure 65. A, If you find the amputated part, rinse it with clean water. **B,** Wrap the part with a dressing and place it in a watertight plastic bag, if it will fit. **C,** Place that bag in another labeled bag that contains ice or ice water.

A

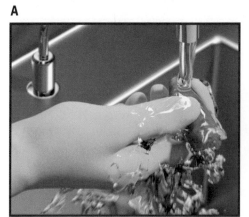

B

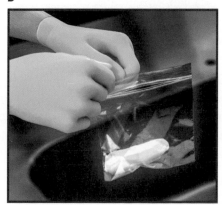

C

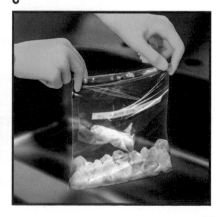

Internal Bleeding

Internal bleeding is bleeding inside the body. When bleeding occurs inside the body, you may be able to see a bruise under the skin, or you may not see any signs at all. When bleeding is internal, you can't tell how much bleeding has occurred.

You should suspect internal bleeding if a person

- Was injured in a car crash or was hit by a car
- Fell from a height
- Was injured in the abdomen or chest (including bruises such as seat belt marks)
- Was injured during a sporting event, such as slamming into other people or being hit with a ball
- Has pain in the abdomen or chest after an injury
- Has shortness of breath after an injury
- Is coughing up or vomiting blood after an injury
- Shows signs of shock without external bleeding
- Was stabbed or shot

Actions to Take: Suspected Internal Bleeding
- Phone 9-1-1, and get the first aid kit and AED.
- If the person is responsive, have the person lie down and keep still while you treat any external injuries.
- Check for signs of shock and provide first aid as needed.
- Be prepared to provide CPR if the person becomes unresponsive and stops breathing normally.

Head, Neck, and Spine Injuries

With any kind of head, neck, or spine injury, be cautious about moving the injured person. Suspect a head, neck, or spine injury if the person

- Fell from a height
- Was injured by a strong blow to the head
- Was injured while diving
- Was involved in a car crash
- Was riding a bicycle or motorbike involved in a crash, especially when not wearing a helmet or when the helmet broke in the crash

A person with a head injury may show these signs:

- Does not respond or only moans
- Acts sleepy or confused
- Vomits
- Has trouble seeing, walking, or moving any part of the body
- Has a seizure

If a person's head injury results in a change in consciousness, worsening signs or symptoms, or other cause for concern, a healthcare provider or EMS personnel should evaluate the person as soon as possible. If the person becomes unresponsive, phone 9-1-1.

A person with these signs should not play sports, drive a car, ride a bike, or work with heavy machinery until a healthcare provider says it's OK to do so.

Concussion

A *concussion* is a type of head injury. Concussions usually happen because of falls, motor vehicle accidents, and sports injuries. A concussion may occur when the head or body is hit so hard that the brain moves inside the skull.

Possible signs of concussion are

- Feeling stunned or dazed
- Confusion
- Headache
- Nausea or vomiting
- Dizziness, unsteadiness, or difficulty in balance
- Double vision or flashing lights
- Loss of memory of events that happened before or after the injury

Spine Injury

Suspect possible spine damage if an injured person

- Is 65 years or older
- Was in a car or bicycle crash
- Has fallen
- Has tingling or is weak in the extremities
- Has pain or tenderness in the neck or back
- Appears intoxicated or not fully alert
- Has other painful injuries, especially to the head or neck

Caution

The spine protects the spine cord, so when a person has a spine injury, do not twist or turn the head or neck unless it's necessary to do any of the following:

- Turn the person faceup to give CPR
- Move the person out of danger
- Reposition the person because of breathing problems, vomiting, or fluids in the mouth

Actions to Take: Possible Head, Neck, or Spine Injury
- Phone 9-1-1 and get the first aid kid and AED.
- Have the person remain as still as possible. Do not twist or turn the person's head or neck unless absolutely necessary.
- Stay with the person until advanced help arrives.

With this type of injury, you may have to control external bleeding. This is why it is important to get the first aid kit. Getting the AED is also important in case the person's condition worsens and you need to give CPR until someone with more advanced training arrives and takes over.

Broken Bones and Sprains

Injuries to bones, joints, and muscles are common.

Signs of Broken Bones

If a person's arm or leg looks deformed after a fall or an accident, a bone might be broken. But other signs of broken bones—such as swelling or bruising, pain when moving, or pain when trying to bear weight—can also be signs of a sprain. Without an x-ray, it may be impossible to tell whether the injury is a broken bone or a sprain. But either way, you'll take the same first aid actions.

Actions to Take: Possible Broken Bone or Sprain

- Put a towel on top of the injured body part. Place a bag filled with ice and water on top of the towel over the injured area (Figure 66). Keep the ice in place for up to 20 minutes.
- The person should avoid using the injured body part until checked by a healthcare provider.
- Phone 9-1-1 if
  - There is a large open wound.
  - The injured body part is abnormally bent.
  - You're not sure what to do.

Figure 66. Put a plastic bag filled with ice and water on the injured area with a towel between the bag and the skin.

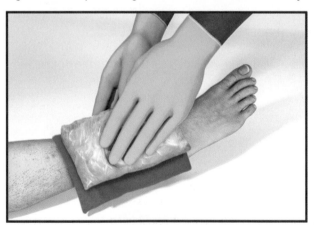

Splinting

A splint keeps an injured body part from moving.

Caution

If the injured part is bleeding, apply direct pressure to stop the bleeding. Apply a dressing to the wound before applying the splint.

Leave bent and deformed body parts in their bent or deformed positions as you apply the splint. If a broken bone has come through the skin, cover the wound with a clean dressing to protect it, and splint as needed.

Actions to Take: Splint

- Find an object that you can use to keep the injured arm or leg from moving.
- Rolled-up towels, magazines, and pieces of wood can serve as splints. Splint in a way to reduce pain and limit further injury. The splint should be longer than the injured area and should support the joints above and below the injury (Figure 67).
- After covering any broken skin with a clean or sterile cloth, secure the splint to the injured limb so that it supports the injured area. Use tape, gauze, or cloth to secure it. It should fit snugly but not cut off circulation.
- If you're using a hard splint, like wood, make sure you pad it with something soft, like clothing or a towel.
- If you don't have anything to use as a splint, have the person place their injured arm across their chest and hold it in place with their other arm.
- Keep the limb still until the injured person can be seen by a healthcare provider.

Figure 67. Use stiff material, such as a stick or a rolled-up magazine, to splint injured body parts.

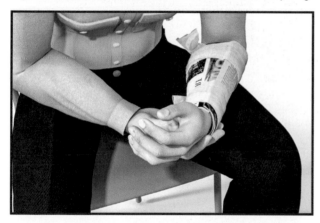

Burns and Electrical Injuries

Burns

Burns can be caused by contact with heat, electricity, or chemicals. Specifically, heat burns are caused when a person comes into contact with a hot surface, hot liquids, steam, or fire.

The only thing you should put on a burn is cool water and clean dressings. Never use ice because it can damage a burned area.

Actions to Take: Small Burns

- Cool the burn area immediately with cold, but not ice-cold, running water for at least 10 minutes (Figure 68).
  - Run cold water on the burn until it doesn't hurt.
  - If you do not have cold water, use a cool or cold, but not freezing, clean compress.
- Cover the burn with a dry, nonstick sterile or clean dressing.
- Follow any further instructions from a healthcare provider.

Figure 68. If possible, hold the burned area under cold running water.

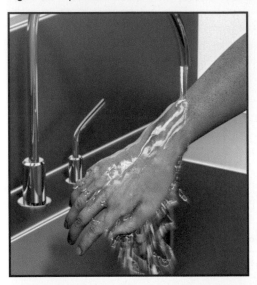

Actions to Take: Large Burns

- If there is a fire, the burn area is large, or you're not sure what to do, phone 9-1-1.
- If the person or their clothing is on fire, put the fire out. Have the person stop, drop, and roll. Then, cover the person with a wet blanket.
- Once the fire is out, remove the wet blanket. Carefully remove jewelry and clothing that is not stuck to the skin.
- For large burns, cool the burn area immediately with cold water for at least 10 minutes.
- After you cool the burns, cover them with dry, nonstick, sterile or clean dressings.
- Cover the person with a dry blanket.
- Check for signs of shock.
- A person with a large burn should be seen by a healthcare provider as soon as possible.
- A healthcare provider can determine if additional treatment is necessary.

Electrical Injuries

Electricity can cause burns on the outside of the body and on the inside, injuring organs. You may see marks or wounds where the electricity has entered and left the body. The damage can be severe, but there's no way to tell how severe by the marks on the outside. Electricity can stop a person from breathing or cause a deadly abnormal heart rhythm and cardiac arrest.

If an electrical injury is caused by high voltage, like a fallen power line, immediately phone 9-1-1. Don't enter the area or try to move wires until the power has been turned off.

Caution

Electricity can travel from the power source through the person to you. Because of this, don't touch an injured person who is still touching the power source. It's best to turn the power off, but only if you are trained to do so. Once the power is off, you can touch the injured person.

Actions to Take: Electrical Injury

- Don't enter the area or try to move wires until the power has been turned off.
- Phone 9-1-1, and get the first aid kit and AED.
- When it is safe to touch the injured person, give CPR if it is needed.
- If the person is responsive, and they have burns or other injuries, treat them.
- A healthcare provider should check anyone who has an electrical injury as soon as possible.

Injury Emergencies: Review Questions

1. To help stop non–life-threatening bleeding that you can see, put firm pressure on a dressing over the bleeding area.
   a. True
   b. False

2. A person with a nosebleed should lean
   a. Forward
   b. Backward

3. If a large stick or a knife has punctured someone's body, you should
   a. Remove it as quickly as possible
   b. Leave it in and get help

4. If someone falls and then becomes sleepy or confused, vomits, or complains of a headache, the person may have a head injury.
   a. True
   b. False

5. If a person twists an ankle, apply a heating pad or heat pack over the injured area for 20 minutes to help reduce swelling.
   a. True
   b. False

6. To give first aid for a small burn on the arm, cool the burn with
   a. Lukewarm water
   b. Ice directly on the skin
   c. Cold, but not ice-cold, water

7. If someone was struck in the abdomen and begins showing signs of shock, suspect internal bleeding.
   a. True
   b. False

8. If someone falls and cuts their leg, you should apply pressure to the nearest pressure point of the leg.
   a. True
   b. False

9. How do you protect an amputated body part?

    a. Place it directly on ice in a sealed bag, and send it to the hospital.

    b. Wrap it in gauze, place it in an airtight bag, and send it to the hospital.

    c. Place it in a watertight plastic bag inside another container with ice or ice and water.

10. If you suspect a concussion, it's OK to let the person play sports until they can see a healthcare provider.

    a. True

    b. False

Answers: 1.a, 2.a, 3.b, 4.a, 5.b, 6.c, 7.a, 8.b, 9.c, 10.b

Environmental Emergencies

For any environmental emergency, your first steps will be to make sure the scene is safe, get the first aid kit, and put on PPE.

Bites and Stings

Animal and Human Bites

When an animal bite breaks the skin, the wound can bleed and become infected. But the bite itself is not the only concern—the person who was bitten might also be at risk for rabies.

Rabies in wild animals is most frequently reported in raccoons, skunks, and bats. Pets bitten by infected animals can become infected. Also, because of the risk of rabies, anyone who has had direct contact with a bat or has even had close exposure to a bat should contact a healthcare provider as soon as possible.

Actions to Take: Animal or Human Bite
- Wash the wound with plenty of soap and water.
- Apply a bag of ice and water wrapped in a towel for up to 20 minutes to help with bruising and swelling.
- For all bites that break the skin, phone a healthcare provider as soon as possible.

Snakebites

Some people can identify a snake from its color or bite mark. But if you're not sure what kind of snake it is, assume that its bite is venomous.

Signs of venomous snakebites are
- Pain at the bite area that keeps getting worse
- Swelling of the bite area
- Nausea, vomiting, sweating, or weakness

Scene Safety and Snakebites

When making sure the scene is safe, be very careful around any snake, even if it's wounded. Back away and go around the snake. If the snake has been killed or hurt, don't handle it. A snake can bite even when severely hurt or close to death.

Actions to Take: Snakebite
- Ask another adult to move any other people away from the area and phone 9-1-1.
- Ask the injured person to stay as still and calm as possible and to avoid moving the part of the body that was bitten.
- Remove any tight clothing and jewelry.
- Gently wash the area with running water and soap.
- Keep the person still and calm until someone with more advanced training arrives and takes over.

Insect, Bee, and Spider Bites and Stings

Usually, insect bites and stings cause only mild pain, itching, and swelling at the bite. However, some insect bites can be serious and even fatal if the person has a severe allergic reaction to the bite or sting or if venom is injected into the person from the bite or sting.

Bees are the only insects that leave behind their stingers. If someone is stung by a bee, look for the stinger and remove it.

> ### Actions to Take: Bite or Sting
> - If the person was stung by a bee, scrape the stinger and venom sac away with something hard and dull that won't squeeze it, like the edge of a credit card or ID card.
> - Wash the sting or bite area with running water and soap.
> - Put a bag of ice and water wrapped in a towel over the area for up to 20 minutes.
> - Watch the person for at least 30 minutes for signs of a severe allergic reaction. Be prepared to use the person's epinephrine pen if needed.

Allergic Reactions to Bee Stings

People who have had severe allergic reactions to an insect bite or sting usually have an epinephrine pen and know how to use it. They often wear medical identification jewelry. If the person develops a severe allergic reaction, phone or send someone else to phone 9-1-1 and get the first aid kit. Use the skills you learned earlier to help the person inject the epinephrine pen.

Venomous Spider Bites and Scorpion Stings

The bite of nonvenomous insects can cause mild signs of redness and itching at the bite area. However, the bite or sting of a venomous spider or scorpion can make someone ill. Signs of venomous spider bites and scorpion stings are

- Severe pain at the site of the bite or sting
- Muscle cramps
- Headache
- Fever
- Vomiting
- Breathing problems
- Seizures
- Lack of response

> ### Actions to Take: Venomous Spider Bite or Scorpion Sting
> - Wash the bite or sting area with lots of running water and soap.
> - Put a bag of ice and water wrapped in a towel on the bite or sting.
> - If you know that a person has been bitten by a venomous spider or scorpion, or if the person has any of these signs after such a bite or sting, they should see a healthcare provider as soon as possible.
> - If the person stops breathing and becomes unresponsive, phone 9-1-1 and start CPR.

Tick Bites

Ticks live in grassy, brushy, and wooded areas, and they attach themselves to exposed parts of the body. Many ticks are harmless, but some carry serious diseases. So if you find a tick, remove it as soon as possible. The longer the tick stays attached to a person, the greater the chance that it will transmit a disease.

Actions to Take: Tick Bite

- Use tweezers to grab the tick by its mouth or head, as close to the skin as possible.
- Try to avoid pinching the tick.
- Lift the tick straight out. If you lift the tick until the person's skin tents and wait for several seconds, the tick may let go.
- Place the tick in a plastic bag so that the person can take it with them when getting medical care.
- Wash the bite area with running water and soap.
- If you are in an area where you know there is tick-borne illness, suggest that the person see a healthcare provider as soon as possible.

Marine Bites and Stings

Just as it's important to be aware of ticks and other insects and animals when you're outside, it's important to be aware of fish and other marine animals when you're in the ocean.

Bites and stings from jellyfish, stingrays, or stonefish may cause pain, swelling, redness, or bleeding. Some marine bites and stings can be serious and even fatal if a person has a severe allergic reaction to the sting or venom.

Actions to Take: Marine Bite or Sting

- Keep the injured person quiet and still.
- Wipe off stingers or tentacles with a gloved hand or towel.
- If the sting is from a jellyfish, rinse the injured area for at least 30 seconds with lots of vinegar. If vinegar is not available, use a baking soda and water solution instead.
- Put the part of the body that was stung in hot water. You can also have the person take a shower with water as hot as they can bear for at least 20 minutes or as long as pain persists.
- Phone 9-1-1 if
  - A person was bitten or stung by a marine animal and has signs of a severe allergic reaction
  - A person was bitten or stung while in an area known to have venomous marine animals
- For all bites and stings that break the skin, see a healthcare provider.

Heat-Related Emergencies

Working, training, or playing in extreme heat can be dangerous. If a person doesn't take the proper care, exposure to extremely hot environments can lead to life-threatening medical conditions.

Dehydration

Dehydration occurs when a person loses water or fluids through heat exposure, too much exercise, illness (such as vomiting, diarrhea, and fever) or decreased fluid intake. Unless it is addressed early, dehydration may lead to life-threatening medical conditions such as shock. Signs of heat-related or environmental dehydration include

- Weakness
- Thirst or dry mouth
- Dizziness
- Confusion
- Less urination than usual

Actions to Take: Dehydration

- If you suspect that a person is dehydrated, contact a healthcare provider right away.
- The best first aid for dehydration is prevention: encourage everyone to drink enough to stay hydrated.

Heat Cramps

Heat cramps are painful muscle spasms, most often occurring in the calves, arms, stomach muscles, and back. Signs of heat cramps are

- Muscle cramps
- Sweating
- Headache

Heat cramps are a sign that heat-related problems may continue to get worse if the person doesn't take action.

Actions to Take: Heat Cramps

- Have the person rest and cool off.
- Have the person drink something with sugar and electrolytes, such as a sports drink or juice, or water if these aren't available.
- If the person can tolerate it, apply a bag with ice and water wrapped in a towel to the cramping area for up to 20 minutes.

Heat Exhaustion

A mild condition, such as heat cramps, can quickly turn into heat exhaustion. That's why it's important to recognize and give first aid for heat-related emergencies early. The signs of heat exhaustion are similar to those of heat stroke:

- Nausea
- Dizziness
- Vomiting
- Muscle cramps
- Feeling faint or fatigued
- Heavy sweating

Actions to Take: Heat Exhaustion

- Have the person lie down in a cool place.
- Remove as much of the person's clothing as possible.
- Cool the person with a cool water spray. If a cool water spray is not available, place cool, damp cloths on the neck, armpits, and groin.
- If the person is responsive and can drink, have the person drink something with sugar and electrolytes, such as a sports drink or juice, or water if these aren't available.

Heat Stroke

Heat stroke is a dangerous, life-threatening condition. So it's important to begin cooling a person who might have heat stroke immediately—every minute counts.

For heat stroke, you should try to immerse the person in cool water immediately. If you can't immerse the person in water, try to cool them with a cool water spray. If the person starts behaving normally again, stop cooling them. If you keep cooling the person, it could lead to low body temperature.

Signs of heat stroke are

- Confusion
- Feeling faint or fatigued
- Dizziness
- Fainting
- Nausea or vomiting
- Muscle cramps
- Seizure

Actions to Take: Heat Stroke

- Phone 9-1-1, and get the first aid kit and AED.
- Move the person from the hot environment, remove any excess clothing they might be wearing, and remind them to limit their physical activity.
- Put the person in cool water up to their neck, if possible, or spray them with cool water.
- If the person becomes unresponsive and is not breathing normally or is only gasping, give CPR.

Cold-Related Emergencies

Frostbite

Frostbite typically occurs outside in cold weather. But it can also occur inside or in a workplace if people are exposed to extremely cold materials, such as cold gases, without wearing gloves. Frostbite affects parts of the body that are exposed to the cold, such as the fingers, toes, nose, and ears.

The signs of frostbite are

- White, waxy, or grayish-yellow skin
- Cold and numb skin
- Hard skin that doesn't move when you push it

Actions to Take: Frostbite

- Phone 9-1-1.
- Move the person to a warm place.
- Remove wet or tight clothing and pat the body dry.
- Put dry clothes on the person and cover them with a blanket.
- Remove tight rings or any bracelets from the frostbitten part.

Caution

- Do not try to thaw the frozen body part if you think there may be a chance of it refreezing before the person can get to medical care.
- Do not rub the frostbitten area. Rubbing may cause damage. If you need to touch the area, do so gently.

Low Body Temperature (Hypothermia)

Hypothermia is another name for low body temperature. Staying too long in a cold, pouring rain or other wet and cold conditions can lead to hypothermia. A person can develop low body temperature even when the outside temperature is above freezing. When hypothermia occurs, it can cause serious problems or even death.

The signs of low body temperature may include

- Skin that's cool to the touch
- Shivering (which stops when the body temperature is very low)
- Confusion
- Personality change
- Sleepiness and the person's lack of concern about their condition
- Stiff, rigid muscles while the skin becomes ice-cold and blue

As the person's body temperature continues to drop, it may be hard to tell if the person is breathing. The person may become unresponsive and might even appear to be dead.

Actions to Take: Hypothermia

- Move the person to a warmer area, remove wet clothing, pat the person dry, and cover with a blanket.
- Phone 9-1-1 and get the first aid kit and AED.
- Put dry clothes on the person.
- Cover the body and head, but not the face, with blankets, towels, or even newspapers.
- Remain with the person until someone with more advanced training arrives and takes over.
- If the person becomes unresponsive and is not breathing normally or is only gasping, give CPR.

Poison Emergencies

A poison is anything that someone swallows or breathes, or that gets into the eyes or on the skin, that causes sickness or death. Many products can poison people.

Poison Control Hotline

The phone number for the poison control center should be in the first aid kit or prominently displayed in areas where chemicals are used. Contact your local poison center by phoning the American Association of Poison Control Centers (Poison Control) at **1-800-222-1222.**

When you phone the Poison Control Center, the dispatcher may ask the following questions:

- What is the name of the poison?
- Can you describe it if you can't name it?
- How much poison did the person touch, breathe, or swallow?
- How old is the person?
- How much does the person weigh?
- When did the poisoning happen?
- How is the person feeling or acting now?

If someone has been exposed to a poison, first make sure the scene is safe. For example, you may need to look for spills of liquids or powders that might be poison.

Actions to Take: Scene Safety in a Poison Emergency

- Look for posted signs warning people that poisons are nearby (Figure 69).
- Look for spilled or leaking containers.
    - If the scene seems unsafe, do not approach. Tell everyone to move away.
    - Stay out of the scene if you see multiple people who may have been poisoned.
- Phone 9-1-1 and get the first aid kit and AED.
- Tell the dispatcher the name of the poison if you know it. Some dispatchers may connect you to a poison control center.
    - Give only those antidotes that the poison control center or dispatcher tells you to. The first aid instructions on the poison itself can be helpful, but they may be incomplete.

Figure 69. Look for symbols of poisons and other hazards, such as these.

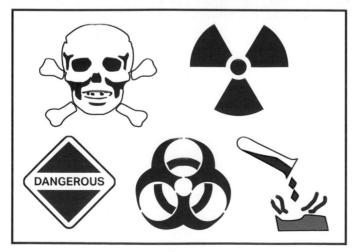

Some places have a safety data sheet (SDS) that provides a description of how a specific chemical or poison can be harmful. It may have first aid recommendations as well. Often, the SDS files are kept in a special binder (Figure 70).

Figure 70. An SDS binder might look like this one.

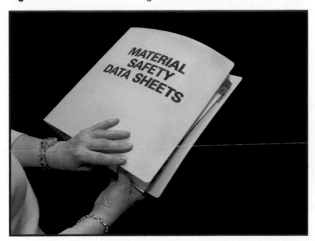

Follow these first aid action steps to remove poison from a person's skin or eyes.

Actions to Take: Poison on the Skin or in the Eyes

- After putting on PPE, move the person from the scene of the poison if you can, and help the person move to an area with fresh air.
- As quickly and safely as you can, wash or remove the poison from the person's skin and clothing. Help the person to a faucet, a safety shower, or an eyewash station.
- Remove clothing and jewelry from any part of the body that the poison touched. Use a gloved hand to brush off any dry powder or solid substance from the person's skin (Figure 71).
- Run lots of water over the affected area until someone with more advanced training arrives and takes over.
- If an eye is affected, ask the person to blink as much as possible while rinsing the eyes. If only one eye is affected, make sure the eye with the poison in it is the lower eye so that you don't rinse the poison into the unaffected eye (Figure 72).
- Give CPR if the person becomes unresponsive and isn't breathing normally or is only gasping. Use a mask for providing breaths. This is especially important if the poison has contaminated the person's lips or mouth.

Figure 71. Brush off any dry powder or solid substances from the person's skin with your gloved hand.

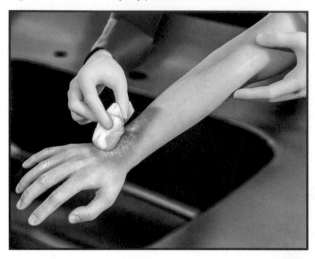

Figure 72. Help the person wash their eyes under water flowing from a faucet or hose, or use an eyewash station.

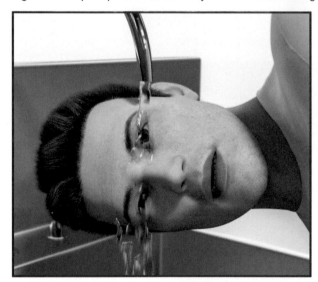

Environmental Emergencies: Review Questions

1. Someone who has been bitten or stung by an insect or bee may have a severe allergic reaction and should be watched for at least _____ minutes.

   a. 10

   b. 20

   c. 30

   d. 60

2. When someone has been bitten, be sure to wash the bite area with a lot of soap and water.

   a. True

   b. False

3. Heat stroke is a life-threatening condition.

   a. True

   b. False

4. If someone was stung by a jellyfish, rinse the area with cold water.

   a. True

   b. False

5. How should you remove a tick?

   a. With a hot matchstick

   b. With lots of alcohol on the skin

   c. By using tweezers

   d. With your hands

6. Being confused may be a symptom of heat stroke and low body temperature.

   a. True

   b. False

7. If you give CPR to someone who has been poisoned, it is important to use a mask, if possible, to give breaths.

   a. True

   b. False

8. When someone has been bitten by a spider, you should

   a. Scrape the spider's fangs away by using something with a dull edge

   b. Remove the victim's clothing, and apply ice directly to the skin

   c. Wash the area with running water and soap

9. For heat exhaustion, spray the person with
   a. A sports drink
   b. Saltwater
   c. Cool water

10. The signs of frostbite are
    a. White, waxy, or grayish-yellow skin
    b. Cold and numb skin
    c. Hard skin that doesn't move when you push it
    d. All of the above

Answers: 1.c, 2.a, 3.a, 4.b, 5.c, 6.a, 7.a, 8.c, 9.c, 10.d

Risks of Smoking and Vaping

The relationship between smoking and lung cancer is well known. But many don't know that smoking is also linked to heart disease, stroke, and other chronic diseases. Smoking can increase your risk for cancer of the bladder, throat, mouth, kidneys, cervix, and pancreas. Let's look at the facts:

- Smoking is a leading preventable cause of death in the United States and globally.
  - About 1 in 5 deaths from heart disease are due to smoking.
  - Smoking is linked to 80% to 90% of lung cancer deaths in the United States.
- Nicotine is a dangerous and highly addictive chemical.
  - It can cause an increase in blood pressure, heart rate, and flow of blood to the heart as well as a narrowing of the arteries or vessels that carry blood.
  - Nicotine may also contribute to the hardening of the arterial walls, which may lead to a heart attack.
  - This chemical can stay in your body for 6 to 8 hours, depending on how often you smoke. Also, as with most addictive substances, there are some side effects of withdrawal.

Today, we are exposed to cigars, cigarillos, e-cigarettes (which can be used for vaping and using a JUUL cartridge), hookah (a type of water pipe), and smokeless tobacco (such as snuff, chew, and dissolvable tobacco). Several of these forms of tobacco are flavored, increasing their appeal, especially to young people. All tobacco products, including smokeless tobacco, hookah, and e-cigarettes, have dangers that include nicotine addiction. Many people falsely believe that e-cigarettes are safe. Some don't even realize they contain nicotine. But they can deliver much higher concentrations of addictive nicotine than traditional cigarettes can.

The bottom line is that tobacco products contain many dangerous toxins. The best thing you can do for your health is to quit tobacco entirely.

You can find resources to help you quit using tobacco products at **heart.org/tobacco**.

How to Quit Tobacco

1 Educate Yourself

The first step to quitting smoking, vaping, and using tobacco is to understand the risks and health effects for you and your family.

➡ **Smoking is the most preventable cause of death in the United States. It's linked to about one third of all deaths from heart disease and 90% of lung cancers.**

➡ **Cigarettes, e-cigarettes, and tobacco products contain many toxic chemicals, as do their smoke, vapor, and liquids.**

➡ **About half of US children ages 3 to 11 years are exposed to secondhand smoke and vapor.**

➡ **Tobacco use and nicotine addiction is a growing crisis for teens and young adults.**

➡ **Within 1 year after quitting, your risk of heart disease goes down by half.**

➡ **You can be one of the millions of people who successfully quit every year.**

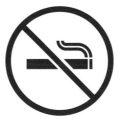

2 Make a Plan to Quit

You're more likely to quit tobacco for good if you prepare with a plan that fits your lifestyle.

Set a quit date within the next 7 days.

Choose a method: cold turkey or gradually.

Decide if you need the help of a healthcare provider, nicotine replacement, or medicine.

Prepare for your quit day by planning how to deal with cravings and urges.

Quit on your quit day.

Learn more at heart.org/Tobacco

3 Tips for Success

 Deal With Urges

Whether physical or mental, learn your triggers and make a plan to address them. Avoid situations that make you want to smoke or use tobacco until you're confident that you can handle them.

 Get Active

Physical activity can help you manage the stress and cravings when quitting. You'll feel better, too. heart.org/MoveMore

 Handle Stress

Learn other healthy ways to manage the stress of quitting. heart.org/BeWell

 Get Support

A buddy system or support program can help you with some of the common struggles of quitting. 1-800-QuitNow

 Stick With It

Quitting tobacco takes a lot of willpower. Reward yourself when you reach milestones and forgive yourself if you take a step backward. Get back on course as soon as possible to stay on track and kick the habit for good.

Benefits of a Healthy Lifestyle

Add Color

Fruits and vegetables provide many beneficial nutrients, including vitamins, minerals, healthy fats, protein, calcium, fiber, antioxidants, and phytonutrients.

On their own, fruits and vegetables typically contain no trans fat, low saturated fat, and very little or no sodium. The natural sugars they contain don't affect your health the same way added sugars do.

Fruits and vegetables also tend to be low in calories, so they can help you manage your weight while still filling you up—thanks to the fiber and water they contain. Replacing higher-calorie foods with fruits and vegetables is an easy first step to a healthier eating plan.

All forms of fruits and vegetables (fresh, frozen, canned, dried, and 100% juice) can be part of a healthy diet. They can be eaten raw or cooked, whole or chopped, organic or not, and alone or in combination with other foods. They are among the most versatile, convenient, and affordable foods you can eat.

A healthy eating plan rich in fruits and vegetables can help lower your risk of many serious and chronic health conditions, including heart disease, stroke, obesity, high blood pressure, high blood cholesterol, diabetes, kidney disease, osteoporosis, and some types of cancer. They're also essential to many daily functions of a healthy body. An easy first step to eating healthy is to include fruits and vegetables at every meal and snack.

To learn more about adding color to your diet, visit **heart.org/addcolor**.

Move More

Here are some tools and tips to get you on the right path to a healthier lifestyle:

- **Just move more!** There are lots of fun and easy ways to build more activity into your everyday routine, even if you're not a gym hero.
- **Set a goal.** Having a commitment or goal, like being active for at least 150 minutes each week, will help you stay on track. Share it with others to keep yourself accountable. If you're the competitive type, challenge friends or family to see who can consistently meet their goals over time.
- **Put fitness first.** Shake up your evening routine. Go for a bike ride or shoot some hoops when you get home from work or school. You'll feel better and think better!
- **Put the screens on hold.** Instead of heading right for the TV or game console after dinner, take a walk or practice a sport.
- **Do what you love.** Find activities that fit your personality and motivate you to stick with them. If you're a social person, try a group dance class or a kickball team, or walk with a group of friends. If you prefer time alone, yoga or running might be a better fit.

For more information, including resources to help you get active, visit **heart.org/movemore**.

Conclusion

Thank you for taking Heartsaver. By learning how to provide first aid and CPR, as well as how to use an AED, you might save a life someday.

Refresh your knowledge by reviewing this book often, and keep the reference guide handy. Even if you don't remember all of the steps exactly, it is important for you to try. Any help is better than no help at all.

More than anything, we want you to have both the knowledge and the confidence to act in an emergency.

Recognizing that something is wrong and getting help on the way are 2 of the most important things you can do.

Join the Nation of Heartsavers™. The AHA wants to recognize the heroes who step in to help save a life during an emergency. If you have a story to share or want to be inspired by other survivor stories, please visit **heart.org/heartsaverhero**.